Strategic Medicines Management

Strategic Medicines Management

Martin Stephens

BPharm, MSc, MRPharmS, MCPP

Chief Pharmacist
Southampton University Hospitals NHS Trust
Southampton, UK

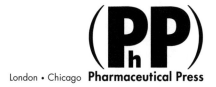

London • Chicago **Pharmaceutical Press**

Published by the Pharmaceutical Press
Publications division of the Royal Pharmaceutical Society of Great Britain

1 Lambeth High Street, London SE1 7JN, UK
100 South Atkinson Road, Suite 206, Grayslake,IL 60030-7820, USA

© Pharmaceutical Press 2005

 is a trade mark of Pharmaceutical Press

First published 2005

Typeset by Type Study, Scarborough, North Yorkshire
Printed in Great Britain by TJ International, Padstow, Cornwall

ISBN 0 85369 598 9

A catalogue record for this book is available from the British Library

For Marjie, Libby and Andy
Thanks for your support

Contents

Preface x
Acknowledgements xi
About the author xii

Introduction   xiii

Medicines and their risks xiii
The emergence of medicines management xiii
What is strategic medicines management? xxii
Does strategic medicines management matter? xxiv
References xxv

1   **National influences**   1

Past policy changes 2
National Institute for Clinical Excellence 8
Medicines advice in Scotland 18
Clinical Resource Efficiency Support Team 19
National Service Frameworks 19
Conclusion 21
References 22

2   **Organisational approaches at a local level**   25

The emergence of drug and therapeutic committees 26
The role of networks 33
The role of the patient and the public 34
A model for drug and therapeutic committees in the modern NHS 35
Conclusion 43
References 43

3   **Formularies**   45

Formularies emerge 45
What kind of formulary? 48
Do formularies work? 52
Developing the evidence base 57
The e-formulary 58
The place of the formulary 59
References 60

4   Managed entry of medicines   63

Why manage entry?   63
A medicine's life cycle   67
Scanning, planning and managing   71
Do we want this new medicine?   74
Evidence-based decisions   76
Conclusion   95
References   95

5   Health economics   99

Economic concepts   100
Economic analyses   104
Critical appraisal of economic analyses   110
Applying health economics   114
The place of health economics   117
References   117

6   Guidelines   121

What are guidelines?   121
The place of guidelines in strategic medicines management   124
How did guidelines emerge?   124
How are guidelines developed and used?   125
Do guidelines work?   133
Legal aspects of guidelines   137
The local approach to guidelines   138
References   140

7   Systematic approaches to strategic medicines management   143

A systematic approach   143
Examples from the literature   144
Shared care arrangements   149
Influencing prescribers   152
Restricting access and saying 'no'   156
Conclusion   160
References   161

8   Managing medicines budgets   163

Horizon scanning and planning   163
Managing budgets in primary care   166
Managing budgets in secondary care   172
Payment by results   175
Conclusion   178
References   178

9   **Performance management**   181

The elements of performance management   182
Applying performance management   187
What targets are there?   188
Making it work locally   192
References   192

10   **The research agenda**   195

Medicines management and pharmacy practice research   195
The NHS context   197
Ethics   199
What are the research questions?   199
The research and development process   204
Funding   206
Conclusion   207
References   208

Index   211

Preface

Medicines play a vital role in the delivery of healthcare; *Strategic Medicines Management* explores the key themes that organisations need to address to get the most from the medicines they use. A National Health Service perspective is taken but the themes of formularies, guidelines and managed entry apply beyond this.

'Medicines management' is a term recently introduced into the realm of healthcare and has been used to mean different things. This text's introduction first explores the term's development and focuses on the organisational aspects, as opposed to individual patient care – only when organisations get strategic medicines management right can patients make the most of their medicines. The main body of the book then deals with the various elements of the subject. Some of the history of these elements is described where appropriate; there is a look at the relevant literature and my own thoughts on how organisations can apply these locally are included.

Strategic Medicines Management is, perhaps, a first attempt to provide, in a single text, a description of an important and evolving subject. Others may wish to include additional themes to the definition provided here, or to challenge the differentiation between the individual and organisational aspects of medicines management. I hope that the book helps this debate and stimulates further work – including practice-based research in this important field.

Strategic Medicines Management is aimed at all healthcare professionals involved in managing medicines in organisations, written by a pharmacist but aimed at the multiprofessional team. It seeks to provide an in-depth introduction to the subject for those with some knowledge of medicines management. It is also a first-time read for those entering this area of work and may be a source of information for more experienced practitioners.

Martin Stephens
February 2005

Acknowledgements

I would like to thank colleagues who have provided advice during the writing of this text. I would also like to acknowledge the reviewers, as I am certain that their comments have improved the content and the style.

About the author

Martin Stephens graduated with a Bachelor of Pharmacy degree from the University of Nottingham in 1979, completing a preregistration year in South Warwickshire hospitals in 1980. He then worked in hospital pharmacy services in the West Midlands region in a variety of posts, becoming Chief Pharmacist at Wolverhampton Hospitals in 1989.

In 1997, Martin became Chief Pharmacist at Southampton University Hospitals NHS Trust, taking on the role of Clinical Director for Clinical Support in 1998. In 2001, he acted as Director of Operations for the trust for a short period before returning to his Chief Pharmacist and Clinical Director role. Martin completed a Masters in health economics and management at Sheffield University in 2000. He is currently chairman of the local area drugs and therapeutic committee and has experience of membership of local and multicentre research ethics committees.

Introduction

Choosing words to mean just what you want them to mean was an approach Lewis Carroll had the scornful Humpty Dumpty declare to Alice.[1] Perhaps this is a hackneyed quotation, but it springs readily to mind when turning to the subject of medicines management. Users of this phrase have certainly chosen their own meaning or held an understanding of it that was clearly at odds with those held by others. Before dealing with the main subject of this text it is important to clarify the term's meaning and that of a few related terms. This introduction attempts to do so and to explore its usage over its relatively short history. It will also examine why the subject is of such importance to healthcare professionals and, indeed, to all users and 'funders' of healthcare.

Medicines and their risks

Medicines are a key part of healthcare; purchasing a medicine or having a medicine prescribed is an event familiar to almost everyone. Medicines may be used as the sole intervention for an acute episode – paracetamol for a headache – or as a continuing therapy in chronic disease – thyroxine for hypothyroidism. They also form the pharmacological arm of more complex interventions, where counselling or lifestyle modification are also sought – antihypertensives. For some non-pharmacological interventions medicines may be required to allow the procedure to take place – anaesthetics. Although commonplace, the use of medicines is a hazardous process, for individuals and for organisations. Adverse reactions, mistakes, misuse, dependence and emerging resistance can have untoward health consequences for individuals and result in significant problems for organisations. The additional concern for organisations is the significant cost of medicines and in particular the burden of continued rapid growth in these costs. The Audit Commission summarises these two features as the risks of medicines, clinical and financial.[2] Dealing with these risks has been a key feature in the process described as medicines management.

The emergence of medicines management

How did the phrase **medicines management**, with its various definitions, come into usage? *The Nuffield Report* of 1986 made no mention of the term, although it did lay out some of the concerns of that time regarding use of the phrase 'clinical pharmacy'.[3] However, the development of clinical pharmacy was supported by the report, and activities that we now call medicines management were clearly described. *The Way Forward* circulars of 1988 lent further support to pharmacy services in NHS hospitals, talking of gaining better care and financial savings by implementing clinical pharmacy.[4] Once again the term 'medicines management' was absent, although the twin themes of clinical and financial benefits were clearly stated.

It is probably helpful to take a sideways step at this point and mention another term that arises in discussion of medicines management: 'pharmaceutical care'. In 1990 Hepler and Strand defined this as 'the responsible provision of drug therapy for the purpose of achieving definite outcomes which improve the patient's quality of life'.[5] This focuses on the individual patient, not at an organisational level; it also raises certain questions: what about interventions that do not improve quality, or those that extend life at reduced quality, or simply protect others or give information? However, the emphasis on the individual does provide an excellent counterbalance to the 'pharmacocentric' approach for which pharmacy has been criticised.[6] Indeed, the United Kingdom Clinical Pharmacy Association (UKCPA), has developed a statement on pharmaceutical care that emphasises this move from 'product orientated custodian' to patient-focused healthcarer.[7] Their statement provides a helpful basis for clinical pharmacy practice, whereas the term 'pharmaceutical care' has itself been revisited and developed, with Cipolle, Strand and Manley's 1998 book identifying its key components.[8]

In the 1990s 'medicines management' also began to emerge as a term, sometimes seen as a rival to 'pharmaceutical care', sometimes seen to supplement that term. At the pharmaceutical conference in 1994 Goldstein and Rivers described their approach to management of medication and encouraged carers to go beyond the therapeutic outcome focus of pharmaceutical care.[9] They described their proposed approach as holistic and suited to working with other healthcarers and social carers. However, they were open to the thought that 'all aspects of medication management' could be the responsibility of informal carers, which suggests their use of this term was not what 'medicines management' is generally understood to mean now.

In the same year Tweedie wrote of 'managing patient therapy', focusing on the need to develop the role of the pharmacist working in community pharmacies.[10] He accepted that many would find

'monitoring patient therapy' a safer phrase because it had less potential to worry the prescriber, whose domain may seem under threat. The
monitor–record–inform general practitioner model he proposed, concentrated on events after receipt of the prescription by the pharmacist;
it was not the more proactive role suggested by pharmaceutical care.
Clinical pharmacy and, more broadly, hospital pharmacy services were
not discussed.

During 1996, 'medicines management' became a regularly used
term, albeit with varied shades of meaning. *The Pharmaceutical Journal*
ran a series of articles under the general title 'medicines management',
although authors did not use the phrase in their texts. The series comprised items describing domiciliary-based medicines review, care home
medicines review, 'brown bag' review in community pharmacies,
primary care clinical guidelines, community-led formulary development
and prescribing analysis and cost (PACT) data.[11–16] Taken together, the
series began to paint a picture of activity encompassing patient specific
and 'population based' roles or services. Hospital pharmacy activity and
roles were not discussed.

The Department of Health launched the National Prescribing
Centre (NPC) in April 1996.[17] Its stated purpose was to facilitate high-
quality, cost-effective prescribing and medicines management. It built on
work undertaken by various other bodies. We will return to its activities
later. At the Pharmaceutical Conference in September that year, Kennard
(Department of Health) emphasised the role of the primary care pharmacist in medicines management and defined the term as: 'facilitating
maximum benefit and minimum risk from medicines for an individual
patient'.[18] She included a more rounded set of activities than had
Tweedie; activities included were optimisation of a patient's regimen,
supply of medicines and monitoring the response. The conference also
saw important initiatives in the hospital service being discussed – the
development of pharmaceutical care and the Scottish plan for a systematic approach to clinical pharmacy.[19]

Adding to the usage of the terminology, Stephens offered a definition of 'medication management' later in 1996.[20] It was used to
describe activities that occur in hospital at a ward level, which might
well be undertaken by pharmacy technicians. Supervision of patients'
own drug schemes, of self-medication projects and general and targeted
counselling were included. Later the term was used in the context of
training for such activities and drug history taking was also included.[21]

Another author, Tomlin, described pharmacy activity as 'managing
medicines', suggesting it had more meaning to the non-pharmacist than

did pharmaceutical care.[22] He did not appear to use the precise definition of pharmaceutical care described earlier in this chapter and he included in his analysis supply of medicines, managing the department and improving patient outcomes.

The proliferation of terms, and the variation in usage of these terms, reflected the development of the profession. Pharmacy had more to offer; as more began to be offered, a new lexicon was appearing.

Keele University's Department of Medicines Management developed out of their Department of Pharmacy Policy and Practice. In 1998 the department's introductory text on medicines management was published. Although the book does not provide a clear definition of the term, the themes addressed are the broader influences and controls on medicines and their prescribing.[24] The ethics of prescribing, economic analyses and systemised controls on prescribing are each addressed. The department's website does provide a definition that supports this inclusive model: 'Medicines management seeks to maximise health gain through the optimum use of medicines. It encompasses all aspects of medicines use, from the prescribing of medicines through to the ways in which medicines are taken or not taken by patients'.[24] This seems a helpful summary, drawing out several aspects for thought, including that health gain is sought, a phrase with health economic tones, and that patients might not take what has been prescribed. Work that could be described as at the 'pre-prescribing' stage, that is formularies and managing new drug entry, isn't mentioned in the definition, although clearly forms a key part of Keele's work.

A different aspect of medicines management came to the fore with the controls assurance programme. During 1999 the NHS Executive began this programme to reduce risk in healthcare. A standard for medicines management was produced.[25] The standard addressed compliance with medicines-related legislation within hospitals; it was received with some disappointment in the service, where medicines management had begun to be seen as more clinically related work, along the lines of Keele's definition. A modified version was released in 2000, which was the basis of the first assessment. It was generally accepted that the standard dealt with an important but limited aspect of a larger subject: safe and secure handling.[26]

Adding to the definitions in the literature, El-Beik and Elliott described medicines management as the promotion of safe, effective and cost-effective medicines usage – usually through policy implementation.[27] Their paper looked at medical staff attitudes to such work, focusing on formularies and guidelines. This was in contrast to the individual patient approach of pharmaceutical care and the Kennard definition of medicines management as described above. Also in 2000, Stephens *et al.* used 'managing medicines' to describe a systematic approach to controlling a hospital drug budget.[28] Chapter 7 develops the theme of an organisational approach that seeks 'good use of medicines' and includes other published work along these lines.

Medicines management had certainly emerged as a term by 2001, although its usage varied. Simpson attempted to clarify the language used on this subject, within a helpful article in 2001: 'What is medicines management and what is pharmaceutical care?' and later in an article in *Pharmacy Management*.[29, 30] The earlier article points out that in most 'English speaking' countries (Simpson includes Scotland), the activities described by the English Department of Health as 'medicines management', are known as 'pharmaceutical care'. Simpson saw the Pharmaceutical Services Negotiating Committee's (PSNC) work in coronary heart disease, also called 'medicines management', as clearly fitting into the Cipolle *et al.* definition of pharmaceutical care.[8] Although acknowledging that there may be medical sensitivities in the use of the term 'pharmaceutical care', he argued that English and Welsh practice should come into line with others. He did not see the terms as synonymous, but rather 'medicines management' as an umbrella term in which pharmaceutical care is included: 'Pharmaceutical care is medicines management but medicines management is not necessarily pharmaceutical care'.

Two others, also in *The Pharmaceutical Journal*, followed this article. Tweedie and Jones noted government documents that sought to move pharmacy forward and suggested that medicines management was an emerging initiative that would develop further etymology.[31] They commented that the Government used 'pharmaceutical care' in a vague sense, although they themselves did not refer to the Hepler and Strand work. Tweedie and Jones defined medicines management as 'the systematic provision of medicines therapy through a partnership of effort between patients and professionals to deliver best patient outcome at minimal cost'. Interestingly they proposed best outcome as cheaply as possible, rather than a more balanced cost-versus-benefits approach, and they focused on the individual rather than on the population. They saw key aspects of medicines management services as 'clinical excellence, collaboration of participants, cost control and concordance'. The discussion was of primary care – community pharmacies, even. Although not specifically excluded, the systematic, whole-health community approach to managing medicines was not addressed.

The second article was from Jenkins and Ghalamkari.[32] Although

Level	Prescription management	Concordance and adherence support	Prescribing policy support	Clinical pharmacy
I	• Dispensing only	• Counselling	• Harmonisation of prescription quantities and rationalisation of strengths	• Ensure clarity and safety of prescription
II	• Collection of prescription from surgery, dispensing and delivery (at request of patient)	• Monitoring of patient requests against patient medication records	• Formulary support	• Monitoring and counselling as per protocol, clinical guideline or integrated care pathway • Clinics for medication review
III	• Instalment dispensing	• Provision of compliance aids	• Empowerment to initiate and manage approved changes in medication	• Pharmaceutical care • Pharmacist prescribing

Increasing intensity (vertical axis, downward)

Increasing integration with other services and level of skills required

Figure I.1 The medicines management matrix. Reproduced with permission from Jenkins and Ghalamkari.[32]

also focusing on primary care services, they provided a helpful analysis of the activities that could be provided under the heading of medicines management. Figure I.1 shows their matrix of services. They agreed with Simpson's analysis that pharmaceutical care is a part of medicines management, holding it up as the better way. However, they acknowledged that patients may not always need the intensive service that pharmaceutical care implies and that other professionals may provide it, while community pharmacists concentrate on other aspects of the service.

During 2001 two important pieces of work related to pharmacy and focusing on medicines management were undertaken for NHS hospitals. The Department of Health issued their medicines management, performance management framework for NHS hospitals in England.[33] The framework identified six areas of activity (domains) that related to

---

Box I.1 Domains in the performance management framework for medicines management.

- Senior management and board awareness and involvement
- Information and financial matters
- Medicines policies including control of drug entry
- Purchasing medicines
- Interface between hospital and primary care
- Influencing prescribers

---

medicine management. These included accountability within organisations, policies and processes. Box I.1 lists these and this, alongside the 2003 update, is discussed in more detail in Chapter 9. The document sought to complement the controls assurance standard, and focused on the clinical and cost-effectiveness aspects of medicines management.

The second piece was the Audit Commission's work within their acute hospitals portfolio. Data were collected from English and Welsh hospital trusts across a range of dimensions, including drug spend and duties undertaken by pharmacy staff. This allowed a form of diagnostic audit, with three areas of enquiry:

- Were there adequate numbers of pharmacy staff, being used for appropriate tasks?
- Were up-to-date practices and processes in place, for example, use of patients' own medicines?
- Was the medicine budget well-managed, that is, not continually overspent by more than a few per cent?

As well as individual feedback to trusts, *A Spoonful of Sugar* was published in December 2001.[2] This was a watershed document, giving a clear definition of medicines management for NHS hospitals: medicines management in hospitals encompasses the entire way that medicines are selected, procured, delivered, prescribed, administered and reviewed to optimise the contribution medicines make to producing informed and desired outcomes of patient care. The document will be discussed throughout the book, but in summary, it dealt with the twin risks – financial and clinical – that medicines pose if medicines management is not done well. It is inclusive, in that it implies work at an individual and organisational level. It could be noted that 'monitoring response' and 'taking' are not included in the definition, and of course the 'not taking' of Keele's definition does not get mentioned in the definition, although compliance (rather than concordance) is discussed in the text. Whilst the focus was secondary and tertiary care, the definition could be applied to a primary care setting.

Within primary care, early in 2001 an important programme led by the NPC was initiated. The national collaborative for medicines management was established, with the first wave of primary care organisations bidding for investment to progress various projects using the collaborative methodology.[34] The programme handbook included a description of the aims of medicines management: 'to prevent, detect and address medicines-related problems and to achieve optimum use of medicines'.[35] Activities were to include advice on prescribing, monitoring and review of medicines, dealing with repeat prescribing and education and training in medicines use. The focus of the work was primary care, but interface issues with hospital care were addressed. Further waves have been established subsequently and in 2004 the first two waves of a similar programme for hospitals was announced.[36]

In 2002 the NPC, jointly with the National Primary Care Research and Development Centre, published *Modernising Medicines Management* as a guide to achieving benefits for patients, professionals and the NHS from these services.[37] Medicines management was defined as a system of processes and behaviours that determine how medicines are used by patients and by the NHS. Thus the individual and organisational aspects of medicines management were included. Five broad groups of service were identified (Box I.2). In 2003 the NPC produced a further document, *PCT Responsibilities Around Prescribing and Medicines Management*, confirming their earlier definition.[38]

Another body that has sought to support those working in medicines management is The College of Pharmacy Practice. In 2001, their Faculty of Prescribing and Medicines Management was established; in the

---

Box I.2 National Prescribing Centre's activity areas in medicines management.

- Clinical – focused on the individual patient
- Systems and processes
- Health of the public – health improvement and risk
- Interface – between primary and secondary/tertiary care
- Patients and their medicines

documents issued, no definition of medicines management was offered (The College of Pharmacy Practice, 2001, personal communication). However, in 2002 a competency framework was launched, which included a mix of patient-focused and organisational-based activities.[39]

In 2002 Simpson again attempted to clarify terminology in the article mentioned earlier.[30] He called for a standard approach:

- Medicines management – an umbrella term along Audit Commission lines.
- Pharmaceutical care – more patient-specific practice along the definition used in the USA.
- Clinical pharmacy – an umbrella term encompassing activities where cognitive, not organisational or commercial, skills are used.

He criticised the diverse approach taken within Britain by the various administrations and made a plea for an educational programme to ensure common ground.

Thus, over a period of around 10 years 'medicines management' has emerged as a term for a range of activities related to choice and use of medicines. There had been a number of attempts to clarify terms, there had been several competing terms, but by 2002–3 a more settled approach had emerged. Hospital pharmacy had taken up the Audit Commission definition, whereas in primary care the initial definition relating to individual patient care activities had been broadened. A broad definition of medicines management has been used by the Department of Health in *Management of Medicines*, published in 2004, where the phrase is defined as including 'the clinical, cost-effective and safe use of medicines to ensure that patients get the maximum benefit from the medicines they need, while at the same time minimising potential harm'.[40]

It is on these broader definitions that this book draws, but having accepted the umbrella term, and at the risk of adding confusion to the terminology, the text concentrates on only part of medicines management. *Hospital Pharmacy* introduced the concept of strategic medicines management – the aspects of medicines management beyond the individual therapy level.[41] The Audit Commission definition is accepted by the text but the strategic elements of influencing the availability of medicines and influencing prescribers are the focus (a hospital perspective is taken). For convenience this group of activity is summarised by the term 'strategic medicines management'. The word 'strategic' is, perhaps, being used nearer its original military meaning: the campaign rather than the tactics; the big picture rather than individual events. Of course in a business context, a strategic approach is seen as the counterbalance of operational management – a strategy seeks to deliver longer-term goals. In medicines management, long-term goals are required by organisations in the way individuals are cared for and in the way that formularies and committees work.

A strategic approach to the issues of medicines management was also highlighted in the Welsh Task and Finish Group; here the importance of clear and transparent decision making on the use of medicines was a key facet.[42, 43]

Figure I.2 attempts to show how the various terms described here interrelate. Medicines management is taken as the broad, overarching term encompassing all activities related to the use of medicines. Pharmaceutical care is taken as the patient-focused aspects – along the lines laid down by Hepler and Strand.[5] Medication management is seen as a part of pharmaceutical care and also going beyond that strict definition, dealing with the practicalities of medication being used by the individuals. Strategic medicines management complements pharmaceutical care as the more organisationally focused elements of medicines management. These are the policies, guidelines and so on, which set the environment in which pharmaceutical care is practised. Finally, clinical pharmacy is placed straddling these domains but not encompassing all, especially as the term implies exclusion of other professions. Medicines management clearly needs all healthcare professionals, patients and carers to contribute, but it is acknowledged that clinical pharmacy is a useful shorthand term for some professional aspects of the whole. (Note that Figure I.2 shows some part of strategic medicines management outside 'medicines management' – somewhat illogical perhaps. The thought behind this is that aspects of strategic medicines management go beyond dealing with medicines and into budget setting and prioritisation related to non-medicines. However, such theoretical discussion is probably of little importance.)

What is strategic medicines management?

Accepting the manufactured nature of the phrase, for the purpose of this book, strategic medicines management is used to describe medicines management activities beyond the level of the individual patient. Figure I.2 divides medicines management into two main parts: pharmaceutical care, dealing with individuals; and strategic medicines management. Box I.3 identifies some of the key elements of strategic medicines management. There are links between the various elements or perhaps blurring of boundaries; an example of this is the overlap between new medicine

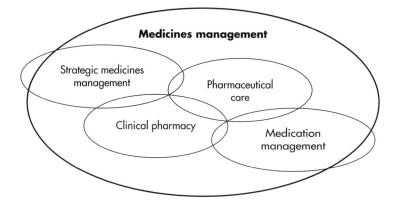

Figure I.2 The elements of medicines management. The diagram has 'medicines management' as the overarching term, which comprises aspects at the individual level and 'strategic medicines management'.

Box I.3 Elements of strategic medicines management.

- Decision-making structures and processes re. medicine usage and policy
- Managing new medicine entry – horizon scanning, planning and managing
- Controlling or steering medicine use – formularies, guidelines
- Managing medicines budgets
- Other influencers of prescribing

---

entry and budgetary control. These activities can also be seen as the layer between national policy and individual patient care. Figure I.3 attempts to summarise this, with strategic medicines management comprising the interpretation of external influences and the setting of local policy. Strategic medicines management's purpose is to produce good medicines use – with reduced clinical risk and sound financial control, attempting to maximise benefits for patients.

Each chapter concentrates on an aspect of strategic medicines management within the NHS. National policy influences throughout the UK are addressed in Chapter 1, including the National Service Frameworks (NSFs) and the National Institute of Clinical Excellence (NICE). How organisations have and should respond is also discussed. Organisation and policy at a more local level is dealt with in Chapter 2; the

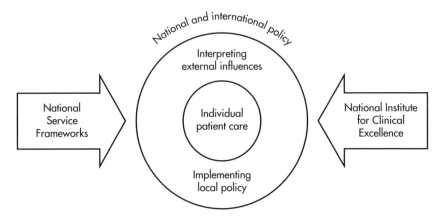

National and international policy

Interpreting
external influences

National
Service
Frameworks

Individual
patient care

National Institute
for Clinical
Excellence

Implementing
local policy

Figure I.3 The place of strategic medicines management: interpreting external influences and implementing local policy.

emergence of drug and therapeutic committees and their role within the current NHS is discussed. Chapters 3–6 deal with some of the tools of strategic medicines management: formularies, guidelines, horizon scanning and assessing the evidence. Chapter 7 looks at the synthesis of these tools in organisations, with some examples of the literature on the subject. Chapter 8 deals with the budgetary aspects of dealing with medicines. Performance management of this key aspect of service is examined in Chapter 9, before a final chapter discussing the research agenda. The book does not examine the important subject of procurement in secondary care, nor is there a detailed discussion of risk management systems, although the latter is touched upon in Chapter 7. Both are important aspects of medicines management and, it could be argued, ought to form part of a discussion of strategic medicines management. However, the boundaries have been drawn around the processes of deciding which medicines should be used, how they might be provided and used in the context of guidelines.

Does strategic medicines management matter?

So far, the evolution of various terms has been described, an evolution that reflects some of development of pharmacy in the past 10 or so years, but why are the elements of strategic medicines management important?

The availability of an enormous arsenal of medicines that carry significant risks in usage and require a large financial commitment has inevitably led to the response of control mechanisms. Ensuring that a regimen suits the individual and that the individual can cope with it, is the obvious level of achieving safe medicines use; this aspect has been excluded from strategic medicines management. However, ensuring that systems are in place and guidance exists in way of policy, formulary and guidelines, are vital mechanisms in supporting individual patient care.

Controlling expenditure is the second aspect of strategic medicines management. This has been an important driver in its evolution. Growth in medicines expenditure has been a feature of the NHS since its inception. During the 1950s the primary care medicines bill grew at around 5% per annum above inflation, Aneurin Bevan is reported to have commented that there seemed no limit to the cascade of medicines going down British throats.[44] Growth in primary care drug spend and in secondary care, where data to monitor have been scarce, has continued and has been met with a variety of responses. Secondary care sought to move costs to general practice – in days before cash limits and single budget streams. Thus discharge length and outpatient supplies were cut, whereas responsibility for prescribing therapies such as erythropoietin and growth hormone were shifted. It could be noted that some of the key tasks of current prescribing and medicines management leads have been to unpick such arrangements!

To choose just a few numbers to illustrate the financial pressure, the total spend in England for primary care prescribing rose from £2858 million in 1992 to £6847 million in 2002 (net ingredient costs quoted).[45] This is an above-inflation growth of 85%, averaging 6.4% per year. This is a very important demand on primary care trust (PCT) resources. In *A Spoonful of Sugar*, secondary care pharmacy services in Wales and England were reviewed and spending growth examined in the period 1998 to 2001.[2] Only four of the trusts showed a fall in spend on medicines, whereas 167 showed growth of up to 60%, with the majority reporting 10–30% growth. This is a crude measure – not accounting for reconfiguration – but hints at the pressure being faced.

Thus both risk to health and risk of financial problems are strong drivers for systematic approaches to strategic medicines management. Done well, financial stability and health benefits are the important outcomes. This text will describe the various elements and look at the evidence of how they contribute to safety, and financial stability approaches that may produce greatest gain will be suggested.

References

1. Carroll L. *Through the Looking Glass*. Chapter 6.
2. Audit Commission. *A Spoonful of Sugar: Medicines Management in NHS Hospitals*. London: Audit Commission, 2001.

3. Clucas K (Chair). *Pharmacy: the Report of a Committee of Inquiry Appointed by the Nuffield Foundation.* London: The Nuffield Foundation, 1986.
4. Department of Health. *The Way Forward for Hospital Pharmaceutical Services* HC 88(54). London: DH, 1988. Also WHC 88(66) (Wales) 1988 and 1988 (GEN) 32 for Scotland 1988.
5. Hepler C, Strand L. Opportunities and responsibilities in pharmaceutical care. *Am J Hosp Pharm* 1990; 47: 533–543.
6. Department of Health. *Pharmacy in the Future.* London: DH, 2000.
7. United Kingdom Clinical Pharmacy Association. UKCPA statement on pharmaceutical care. http://www.ukcpa.org/default.asp?channel_id=447& editorial_id=1819 (accessed 8 December 2004).
8. Cipolle R, Strand L, Marley P. *Pharmaceutical Care Practice.* New York: McGraw-Hill, 1998.
9. Goldstein R, Rivers P. Pharmaceutical care: a new approach to the management of medication by elderly people. *Pharm J* 1994; 252: R14.
10. Tweedie A. Managing patient therapy. *Pharm J* 1994; 252: 507–508.
11. Beech E, Brackley K. Domiciliary based medication review for the elderly. *Pharm J* 1996; 256: 620–622.
12. Sommerville H. Medication review in nursing and residential homes. *Pharm J* 1996; 256: 648–650.
13. Goodyear L, Lovejoy A, Nathan A, Warnett S. 'Brown bag' reviews in community pharmacies. *Pharm J* 1996; 256: 723–725.
14. Hardy N. Developing and implementing clinical guidelines in primary care. *Pharm J* 1996; 256: 757–759.
15. Jenkins A. Formulary development by community pharmacists. *Pharm J* 1996; 256: 861–863.
16. Bevan B. PACT data avoiding the pitfalls. *Pharm J* 1996; 257: 25–30.
17. Anon. The National Prescribing Centre: encouraging high-quality practice. *Pharm J* 1996; 257: 282–285.
18. Anon. A role for pharmacists in medicines management. *Pharm J* 1996; 257: 418.
19. Anon. Developing pharmaceutical care. *Pharm J* 1996; 257: 414–415.
20. Stephens M. To where should the role of the pharmacy technician extend? *Pharm Pract* 1996; 6: 406.
21. South East Medicines Management Education Team. Medication management accredited course for pharmacy technicians. http://www.pharmacyet.co.uk (accessed 8 December 2004).
22. Tomlin M. Value analysis of hospital pharmaceutical services – pharmacy: expensive or valued. *Pharm Manage* 1998; 14: 2–4.
23. Panton R, Chapman S, eds. *Medicines Management.* London: BMJ Publishing Group and Pharmaceutical Press, 1998.
24. Keele University Department of Medicines Management. http://www.keele.ac.uk/depts/mm/General/index.htm (accessed 13 December 2004).
25. NHS Executive. *Medicines Management Controls Assurance Standards.* London: NHSE, 1999.
26. Department of Health. *Medicines Management (Safe and Secure Handling).* London: DH, 2000.

27. El-Beik S, Elliot R. Exploring hospital clinicians' view of medicines management. *Pharm J* 2000; 265: R61.

28. Stephens M, Tomlin M, Mitchell R. Managing medicines: the optimising drug value approach. *Hosp Pharm* 2000; 7: 256–259.

29. Simpson D. What is medicines management and what is pharmaceutical care? *Pharm J* 2001; 266: 150.

30. Simpson D. Making sense of medicines management. *Pharm Manage* 2002; 18: 56–58.

31. Tweedie A Jones I. What is medicines management? *Pharm J* 2001; 266: 248.

32. Jenkins D, Ghalamkari H. A pragmatic way forward. *Pharm J* 2001; 266: 281.

33. Department of Health. *The Performance Management of Medicines Management in NHS Hospitals.* London: DH, 2001.

34. National Primary Care Development Team. National Prescribing Centre Collaborative methodology. http://www.npdt.org/scripts/default.asp?site_id= 1&id=367 (accessed 8 December 2004).

35. National Prescribing Centre. *Collaborative Medicines Management Services Programme Handbook.* Liverpool: NPC, 2001.

36. Hospital Medicines Management Collaborative. http://www.npc.co.uk/mms/ hmmc/index.htm (accessed 8 December 2004).

37. National Prescribing Centre and National Primary Care Research and Development Centre. *Modernising Medicines Management.* Liverpool and Manchester: NPC and NPCRDC, 2002.

38. National Prescribing Centre. *PCT Responsibilities Around Prescribing and Medicines Management.* Liverpool: NPC, 2003.

39. Faculty of Prescribing and Medicines Management. *A Competency Framework for Members and Associates.* Coventry: College of Pharmacy Practice, 2002.

40. Department of Health. *Management of Medicines.* London: DH, 2004.

41. Fitzpatrick R. Strategic medicines management. In Stephens M, ed. *Hospital Pharmacy.* London: Pharmaceutical Press, 2003.

42. National Assembly for Wales. *Report Of the Task and Finish Group on Prescribing.* Cardiff: National Assembly for Wales, 2000.

43. Anon. Pharmacist picked to lead influential medicines strategy group in Wales. *Pharm J* 2002; 209: 316.

44. Klein R. *The New Politics of the NHS*, 3rd edn, London: Longman, 1995.

45. Department of Health. *Statistical Bulletin 2003/12: Prescriptions Dispensed in the Community Statistics 1999–2002, England.* London: DH, 2003.

1

National influences

Strategic medicines management can be viewed as the filling in the sandwich between national policy and individual patient care. It sets the local policy framework and applies external influences in a local context. This chapter examines a few historical influences on strategic medicines management, then explores a selection of the current key features, including the role of the National Institute for Clinical Excellence (NICE).

Selecting which are the current most pertinent influences is difficult; deciding which have been the most influential over the past 30 years or so is almost impossible. Society has changed in many ways, including in attitudes to health and healthcare; there have been significant demographic changes; laws regulating medicines have changed; many more therapeutic options have become available and new prescribers have emerged. Each of these elements has consequences for organisations and shapes their strategic medicines management response. The way the pharmaceutical industry develops and markets medicines and how they are regulated are also important influences. Control of pharmaceutical profits, the way research investment is treated, law relating to clinical trials and the organisation of research ethics committees also have influence.

An important societal change that has relevance to medicines use could be described as a move away from a 'paternalistic' approach to prescribing – the professionals knowing best, albeit completely committed to doing the best for their patients. Labels stating 'the tablets' or 'the mixture' rather than the product's name, with no thought of a patient information leaflet, and issued with the instruction to follow the doctor's orders, used to be commonplace. We now have a growing commitment to the individual consumer-focused approach, with patient empowerment seen as vital. This shift changes the environment in which strategic medicines management is delivered. Patients are well-informed and are prepared to contest decisions regarding access to medicines. Rightly, patients have recourse to law where decisions are taken to limit access to medicines. This means that due care and proper procedure should be adhered to by organisations seeking to manage medicines. Indeed, organisations and individual healthcare professionals should seek to reap the benefits of the empowerment and involvement of patients, not see it as an inconvenience. Good decisions about the availability of medicines, and use of medicines according to best evidence are of no value if the potential recipient is not going to take those medicines. Perhaps seeing the patient as an informed partner in prescribing decisions is the way to develop concordance and avoid waste. Certainly the move to empowerment rather than paternalism is seen as here to stay and as providing opportunity to improve self-care.[1,2]

These social and cultural changes are important. Although the chapter concentrates on policy decisions in the main, these policies themselves could be seen as driven by societal changes. The chapter does not seek to deal with all national influences, but later in the book the influence of the Department of Health, the Audit Commission and other bodies on specific aspects of strategic medicines management will be addressed.

Past policy changes

The prescription charge

In 1952 the UK government introduced a modest co-payment of one shilling for each National Health Service (NHS) prescription dispensed. Although politically controversial, the aim was to offset the growing costs of the service, by then in its fifth year, and to dampen the increasing demand. In 1956 the charge moved from a per prescription to a per item basis and in 1961 it was increased to two shillings. The 1965 Wilson government abolished charges only to reintroduce them in 1968 at two shillings and sixpence (equivalent to 12.5p) per item. However, in 1968, exemptions for children, the low paid and the elderly were introduced. Further exemptions on health grounds were introduced in the 1970s, during which period the charge remained stable at 20p per item. During the era of the Thatcher government from 1979 to 1990 the charge rose from 20p to £3 and by 1993 was at £4.25. This has been calculated as equivalent to a 750% increase after allowing for inflation.[3] Further rises throughout the 1990s and into the 21st century have taken the fee to over £6 per item, but with a wide range of medical and income-related exemptions, as well as age- and pregnancy-related exemptions. Although not strictly relevant to the prescription fee level, over the 1990s the net ingredient cost per item rose from about £6 to about £10.

Since devolution within the UK, some variation has occurred in the exemption categories. In addition, a number of types of prescriptions are exempt from fees, such as those for the oral contraceptive and items from a sexually transmitted disease clinic. By 2002 it was estimated that around 50% of the population in England were eligible for free prescriptions and during 2002 only 14% of items dispensed by community pharmacists incurred a fee.[4] Hospital outpatient, but not discharge, prescriptions also require fee collection, and guidance also exists for day surgery patients to be charged.[5]

In the context of strategic medicines management, the key question is whether prescription charge policy has an impact on demand. Ryan and Yule examined this in 1993, noting that there are three possible ways demand could be reduced.[3] These were by deterring consultation with a doctor; by discouraging the demand for prescriptions at consultation; and by discouraging patients from having the prescriptions dispensed. They concluded that charge introduction, charge increase and reintroduction each had an impact on the number of prescriptions dispensed and that co-payment did indeed reduce demand.

Beardon *et al.* provide further evidence that supports the negative effect prescription charges have on demand: they found that non-exempt patients are less likely to get their prescription dispensed than those exempt from charges.[6] This they described as primary non-compliance. Of course, where prescribed items are available via sale it may be that the informed patient or, under guidance of the pharmacy staff, anyone may choose to purchase the item if costs are less than the prescription fee. Freemantle and Bloor looked at the international experience on co-payments and concluded that they do indeed reduce medicine use, both of desirable medicines and those considered less desirable.[7] Schafheutle expressed concern that the impact that charges have on uptake of 'desirable' medicines could lead to increased morbidity and mortality, and set out to investigate who is most at risk from these cost-controlling personal decisions.[8] If this is the case, then a vital question for policy makers is whether the extra costs of dealing with the increased morbidity outweighs any savings from reduced demand plus any revenue raised.

Many have argued for changes in the way charges are administered: removing or increasing exemptions, and so on. In 1998 Professor Walley suggested an 'effectiveness model for charges', the top 200–300 medicines being free to all, those medicines with little extra benefits or costly extra benefits to have a modest co-payment, then items such as branded generics requiring 50% of the cost to be charged.[9] Such a model has not been proposed by the Department of Health.

Individual organisations must live with the current system of charges. It is difficult to see how an organisational response or policy can be developed to ensure that the impact of charges is managed, but it would seem wise not to ignore the subject. Individual prescribers will be aware of the circumstances of each patient, and considering strategies to avoid multiple charges may support good medicine use. Use of combination products would support this for patients who pay, although there may be other reasons to avoid such combinations – premium pricing and fixed dose ratios. Length of supply could also be used to reduce costs for payers but again there are good reasons for giving a standard, not excessive, length of supply for reasons of equity and to avoid waste, respectively. It may be that a negotiation with the paying patient about which items they could do without is the pragmatic approach to take, perhaps undertaken by the pharmacist rather than the general practitioner. Using pre-payment certificates to cover all items, where this is worthwhile, can of course be a method of overcoming the 'Which do I choose?' dilemma. Overall, those involved in medicines management need to be aware of the potential impact of prescription charges on medicine use, even if there is little that can be done to influence that impact.

The limited list

The limited list of NHS medicines was introduced in 1985 with the aim of restricting the availability of NHS-prescribed medicines to those 'necessary to meet all clinical needs' but where those needs could be met 'at the lowest possible cost to the NHS'.[10] A range of antacids, laxatives and minor ailment reliefs became non-prescribable on the NHS. Additionally benzodiazepines became prescribable only by generic name or in specific circumstances. The current *British National Formulary* indicates these non-prescribable products by the specific symbol of the letters NHS in a box with a diagonal line through it.[11] The aim was to save around £75 million from the national medicines budget, although it was disputed if such savings did occur.[3] The suggested main reason for failing to make savings was the substitution effect – moving from a cheap, ineffective, prohibited medicine to a more expensive, slightly more effective, permitted medicine increases cost. Yule *et al.* noted there may have been reduced effectiveness and a shift to patients paying for medicines themselves.[12]

As with prescription charges, those responsible for strategic medicines management can do little in response to the limited-list policy, other than note its presence. In 1985 its arrival was seen as an important challenge to clinical freedom; its impact was probably of limited long-term significance. Further extension of the list was considered but not pursued. The combined pressures of industry and those wishing to retain clinical freedom, as much as the evidence of lack of impact, meant no further steps were taken.

The NHS funding flows

Although not a direct influence on medicines use, the way NHS organisations receive funds has affected strategic medicines management. Until the post-1997 NHS reforms, health authorities received two types of funding allocation: hospital and community health services (HCHS) funds and general medical services (GMS) funds. Put simply, HCHS funds were used to pay for hospital care, whereas GMS funds included a non-cash-limited allocation for primary care dispensing. Although changes were made during fundholding (see next section), the most significant change occurred with the white paper *The New NHS – Modern, Dependable* in 1997.[13] This introduced a 'single stream of funds' for health authorities, and later for primary care organisations, meaning both the hospital costs and the prescription costs came out of the same pot. The historical 'blank cheque' of the general practice prescription had suddenly been linked to the funds available for hospital care. Overspend on prescribing could result in a reduction in funds available for hospital care; such a risk concentrated the minds of hospital managers and many clinicians. It also brought an opportunity to think as a health community – if not with a single budget for medicines, at least a single source of funding.

During the years before the change in funding flow, there was a great temptation to shift costs from secondary care to primary care, from a cash-limited budget to the open-ended primary care pot. Specialist, high-cost medicines were moved to primary care from hospitals – erythropoietin in renal medicine being one example. Crump *et al.* described some of the issues in 1995.[14] They examined the use of several high-cost medicines in the West Midlands Region, reporting spend in primary and secondary care. For example, whereas growth hormone spend in secondary care was just under £250,000, it was over £2 million in primary care. Cyclosporin, fluids for continuous ambulatory peritoneal dialysis, erythropoietin, recombinant human deoxyribonuclease and risperidone were also discussed, each being a medicine initiated by a hospital specialist but where primary care physicians were undertaking the majority of the prescribing. They pointed out that this 'back door' access to funds might mean that the benefits of new, expensive medicines were not considered, whereas in hospitals, use was far more rigorously examined. In effect, the ability to move out specialist prescribing avoided the rationing decisions being applied to other aspects of secondary care. Shared care prescribing will be explored later in this text, but the point Crump and others have made is that complex therapy, requiring specialist monitoring, ought to have remained with the specialist; finances meant such prescribing moved to general practice.

Another aspect of cost shifting was that hospitals reduced the length of supplies for discharge and outpatient prescriptions. Although there is no single 'right' way to provide such services (for example, Scotland and England have quite different models for outpatient medicines), changes were again made to reduce costs in hospitals rather than because a preferred model of care had been found. Bringing all the costs into a single cash-limited flow of funds (now via primary care trusts for England) means that cost shifting is no longer attractive. Organisations and the health community can explore who is the most appropriate prescriber of a medicine rather than playing a game of 'dodge the budget control'. Likewise, original pack supply can be encouraged rather than a few tablets provided at discharge. The key questions become: what is best for the patient and does the prescriber have the appropriate knowledge? Cost may have an influence, particularly where hospital discounts and value-added tax differences are relevant, but this does not need to be the over-riding factor.

Moving to a unified approach to budgets is not without its critics. The tempting, unrestricted, primary care purse used by hospitals in the early 1990s clearly needed to be addressed. However, financial pressures on other parts of primary care organisations' budgets could mean that any savings in prescribing budgets would be swallowed up. Rao made this point based on local experience – reporting that the use of prescribing savings to assist the cost pressures on the acute trust provider caused general practitioners to feel they had wasted their efforts.[15] This issue is real but needs to be overcome; it can be a recurring theme in any complex organisation where areas of good performance may end up compensating for areas of concern of poor control.

General practice – fundholding and incentive schemes

The idea of a non-cash-limited budget for medicines has been raised. However, it would be wrong to leave the impression that no effort was being made to control spending before the change in funding flows. Indicative prescribing budgets and prescribing reviews were already in place and with the introduction of fundholding practices in the early

1990s, some general practitioners in effect had their own cash-limited prescribing budgets. The impact has been examined by a number of authors. Harris and Scrivener analysed national data for all general practices in England over the six years from April 1990 to 1996.[16] They discovered that the absolute cost of prescribing increased greatly across all practices but to a slightly lesser degree in fundholders. Interestingly, the relative reduction in costs of fundholders, compared with non-fundholders, began in the pre-fundholding year and reached about 6% over the first three years of fundholding. However, they also noted no further gains were made. Reduction in costs was achieved by reduction in the average cost per item rather than by decrease in the number of items dispensed. They concluded that, in financial terms, fundholding had been a success. Wilson *et al.* confirmed this in one UK region in their report of 1997.[17] Baines *et al.* compared fundholding with indicative prescribing budgets schemes in rural practices and again confirmed the benefits of fundholding with respect to costs.[18]

Changes in budget responsibility may result in greater engagement of clinicians, in any sector; when the fundholding schemes were wound up in the 1997 reforms, new systems were required. In 1999 primary care organisations were required to have prescribing incentive schemes. The schemes started in 1999 were thought to be an improvement on the drivers in fundholding since, under incentive schemes, quality as well as cost could be encouraged. Work undertaken by Ashworth *et al.* found that many primary care organisations included both cost and quality features in their schemes and that there were improvements in quality indicators.[19,20] Sullivan gave a rather more sceptical view on the findings, noting the confounding factors, such as extra pharmacist input, although perhaps pharmacist input itself was a result of the incentive scheme.[21] Certainly the NPC includes continuing with incentives for high-quality prescribing as a key aspect of financial management for primary care trusts (PCTs).[22]

Although fundholding is no longer a feature, the local strategic medicines manager will need to be aware of, and to work with, the budgetary and incentive arrangements to achieve best use of medicines. Chapter 8 gives more space to budget management in primary and secondary care organisations.

Medicines for sale

Before moving to some of the current national bodies affecting medicines management, it is worth noting that medicine use is influenced by the availability of over-the-counter medicines – general sales products and those restricted to sale by a pharmacist. The sale, rather than supply, on prescription was noted earlier in the context of prescription charges. The idea of deregulation having an impact on prescribing costs is explored briefly in *Medicines Management*.[23] The conclusion was that there is little evidence to suggest increasing the availability via sale of medicines has an impact on the demand for GP appointments, but that there is evidence of a preference to purchase rather than paying prescription charges. The availability of aspirin and statins without pre-scription – one relatively cheap, the other more costly – might increase access to cardiovascular protection, but it is not clear that this will have a significant impact on medicines management in primary care organis-ations. A watching brief and awareness of the issue is probably the best approach.

National Institute for Clinical Excellence

In 1997 the newly elected Labour government introduced an important white paper that announced a wide range of changes, including the abolition of fundholding already mentioned.[13] In Section 7 of the docu-ment, a new National Institute for Clinical Excellence (NICE) was described. It was to be established to produce and disseminate clinical guidelines based on relevant evidence of clinical- and cost-effectiveness, associated audit methodology and information on good practice. One of the key drivers for NICE was the desire to see consistent delivery of care across the National Health Service – 'no more postcode prescribing' was the headline. *A First Class Service* was published later and provided further details on how NICE would work.[24] NICE was set up as a Special Health Authority in April 1999 with board and staff, to under-take the various streams of work. The stated aim was to assist doctors, nurses, midwives and other healthcare professionals to provide the most effective treatments, while also protecting patients from ineffective care. The arrival of NICE was greeted with a positive editorial in the *British Medical Journal* in March 1999.[25] The role of assessing new technolo-gies was seen as the early focus and welcomed as an explicit national approach to rationing, replacing the rather chaotic way access to medi-cines had been evolving. However, Smith was concerned that the work on guidelines would be less useful in that 'centralist direction is a poor way of solving' variability in practice.[25]

At the time of writing, Professor Sir Michael Rawlings is the Chair and Andrew Dillon is the Chief Executive; as well as the experts working on specific projects, NICE has a 30-member strong Citizens' Council.[26] NICE provides advice for England and Wales in three ways: clinical guidelines, interventional procedure guidance and technology appraisals.

The clinical guidelines issued by NICE include those inherited but endorsed (such as the 2001 issue of myocardial infarct prophylaxis) and those newly commissioned (such as the 2003 head injury guideline).

Technology appraisals

The first two technology appraisals dealt with wisdom teeth removal and hip prostheses (these can be found in summary in the compilation books[27]). Appraisal number 3 dealt with taxanes in ovarian cancer, this version was replaced in January 2003 by assessment number 55.[28] Appraisal numbers 77 and 79 were issued in April 2004, the most recent at the time of writing; these dealt with 'the z-drugs' in insomnia, and newer epilepsy medicines in children respectively.[29,30]

Technology appraisals follow an agreed process of production; this is summarised in the NICE compilation documents or is available via the website.[26,27] Technologies are selected where they meet one or more of the following criteria:

- Is there likely to be a significant health gain from the intervention?
- Will there be a significant health gain impact on government policy aspirations, such as reducing health inequalities?
- Will there be a significant impact on resources?
- Will NICE help resolve a controversy over the evidence on clinical or cost effectiveness?

The process of appraisal, from selection to use, is summarised in Figure 1.1. The assessment report is a key part of this process, where evidence is critically appraised, including clinical and health economic data. The Appraisal Committees include clinicians, managers, patient advocates, industry representatives and academics, all chosen from a panel and supplemented by specific 'experts' that have first-hand knowledge of the technology being appraised. Industry, and others, have the opportunity to appeal against the guidance at the consultation stage; a formal appeals process is followed when this occurs. If the appeal fails and where no appeal is lodged, the consultation document becomes the final guidance. The guidance may support the technology freely, provide caveats to use, advise that it should only be used in a trial setting or advise that it should not be available via the NHS. Clearly, the final

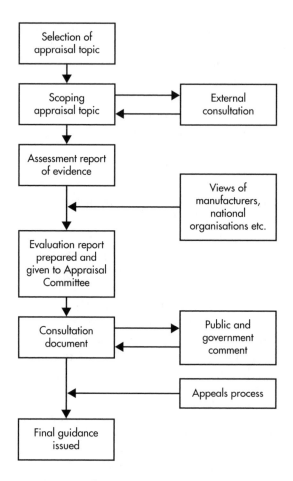

Figure 1.1 National Institute for Clinical Excellence technology appraisal.

category provides bad news for the manufacturer who will have made significant investment to get the product to market and as such would probably have been subject to vigorous challenge at the appeal stage. Patient groups and clinicians may also have concerns where treatments expected to bring big benefits are restricted. The less partial observer may reflect that conserving resources for the more clinical and cost-effective interventions, rather than for the NICE 'rejected' technology is in the best interests of the whole population, as those resources are finite.

A case which received considerable attention was the guidance issued by NICE on interferon beta and glatiramer acetate for multiple sclerosis.[31] The guidance was that, on the balance of clinical and cost-effectiveness, neither therapy should be available on the NHS in

England or Wales. To avoid problems it was proposed that patients already receiving therapy should be given the option of continuing. Even before the final guidance was issued there was considerable concern expressed (in late 2000). This comment was described as a barrage of criticism and included statements from the Multiple Sclerosis Society; the Association of British Neurologists also made a plea for free access to these medicines.[32] The NICE appraisal did suggest that there were ways of making the treatment available 'in a manner that could be considered cost-effective', and a risk-sharing scheme subsequently allowed this to be taken forward. Discussions with the suppliers to manage the price were undertaken in the scheme's development.

A further incident in 2000 resulted in a critical *British Medical Journal* editorial regarding the zanamivir appraisal (number 15).[33,34] The processes were much criticised as was the guidance. Rawlins provided a robust defence restating the purpose of NICE and emphasising the independence of the appraisal process.[35] NICE had supported zanamivir's use, whereas many clinicians felt this was not justified by the evidence.

A more measured criticism of NICE arrived in September 2001.[36] Taking an economist's perspective, Cookson, McDaird and Maynard argued that NICE needed to be less supportive of new technologies and to say 'no' more often. To support new technologies continually would, they said, cause investment to move away from other services to support NICE-approved therapies – at the expense of the overall health of the community. Although reasoned well, the article also stated, rather emotively: 'Instead of challenging the pharmaceutical industry to show value for money, NICE has become their "golden goose" '!

In 2002, Dent and Sadler produced a review of NICE outputs.[37] They contrasted NICE support for technologies with advice from other reviewers, where those others had not favoured use. They also noted the paucity of evidence on which some decisions were based. Within the discussion they suggested that NICE had much broader acceptance criteria that other evaluation groups. One conclusion that could be drawn by the reader is that, traditionally, evaluation committees needed to be convinced of the worth of a medicine before offering support, whereas NICE needs to have strong reasons *not* to support a licensed medicine's availability on the NHS.

A topic of debate since the inception of NICE has been the question of a cost-effectiveness threshold. Chapter 5 visits this in the context of health economics, but the essence of the question is whether there is or should be a fixed 'value for money' point beyond which technologies are not supported. The suggestion has been made that a technology costing more than £30,000 per quality-adjusted life year would not be supported. The chairman of NICE has strongly denied this rule is followed; Towse, Pritchard and Devlin discuss the proposition and evidence in detail in *Cost-effectiveness Thresholds* and give examples of NICE support for technologies above the £30,000 mark.[38] NICE has rejected technologies across a range of cost-effectiveness levels, restricted others but accepted the majority of items reviewed.

Initially, NICE recommendations had the legal status of guidance, to be considered carefully but were not obligatory.[33] From 2002, English primary care trusts had a statutory obligation to provide appropriate funding to support technology appraisal guidance within three months of guidance being issued – unless a specific extension is permitted. There is therefore a real pressure to ensure that guidance is implemented, even if at the expense of other programmes seen as priorities locally.

Technology appraisals are regularly produced, revised when necessary and demand the attention of primary and secondary care organisations. They aim to deliver a consistent approach to new technologies and to reduce delays in access to new medicines.

NICE clinical guidelines

The first of the inherited clinical guidelines was issued by NICE in April 2001.[39] It dealt with drug treatment, cardiac rehabilitation and dietary manipulation in secondary prevention of myocardial infarcts. The technology appraisals examine a specific intervention or group of related interventions, answering the question whether it should be available on the NHS. The clinical guidelines give healthcare professionals and patients broader guidance on the care and interventions to be used in a particular situation. The various aspects of care are graded on a scale to indicate the confidence level in the evidence used to support the advice. Thus the myocardial infarct guideline gives the top grade (A) of support for use of aspirin but a lower grade for the start point for a statin as there is less certainty on the appropriate cholesterol level to initiate therapy. Chapter 6, on guidelines, explores the approach taken to levels of supporting evidence.

The first of the newly commissioned clinical guidelines was produced in December 2002, dealing with care interventions in schizophrenia.[40] It was developed by the National Collaborating Centre for Mental Health. In parallel with the technology appraisal on atypical antipsychotics, the guideline recommended oral atypical antipsychotics as the first choice in treatment of newly diagnosed cases of schizophrenia.

As with technology appraisals, clinical guidelines produced by NICE can be drivers in ensuring access to therapies that are supported by the evidence, yet have been considered unaffordable, or are just not commonly used. Their more complex nature, bringing a long series of recommendations, mean they require more attention and effort from local organisations than the more straightforward technology appraisals.

The first step in guideline development by NICE is to describe a topic and to seek expressions of interest from stakeholders. This would include professional bodies and patient groups. Each topic is then developed by one of the seven National Collaborating Centres, listed in the NICE compilation books.[27] Each centre focuses on a particular area of work, for example, cancer or chronic conditions. Scoping is undertaken by the relevant centre and details are provided for consultation with the stakeholders. The scoping document will include the list of consultees, which treatments are to be included and the method of assessing cost effectiveness. The draft and comments received are examined by one of NICE's independent Guideline Review Panels. These panels replaced the original Guidelines Advisory Committee in 2003. Scoping over, the centre sets up a guideline development group to undertake the review of the evidence and the collation of the guideline. After various drafts and consultations NICE publishes the validated guideline.

NICE-inherited and newly commissioned guidelines have probably been far less controversial than the technology appraisals. However, there have been concerns raised about them. Wailoo *et al.* make several interesting points.[41] The thrust of their argument is that, unlike technology appraisals, NICE guidelines fail to consider cost-effectiveness appropriately in making recommendations. They argue that reliance on strength of evidence and on the fact that development groups comprise clinicians with a particular interest, plus patient representatives, tend to produce a wish list of interventions rather than balanced advice on efficient and equitable use of resources. This will require time to be judged fairly.

A more broadly based concern regarding guidelines is that just producing a document does not in itself change practice. Chapter 6 develops this topic further. Even so, the availability of nationally developed and endorsed guidelines does assist local organisations in their efforts to ensure evidence-based medicine use.

How is NICE doing?

At a meeting around the launch of NICE, the chairman was asked if NICE was an evidence-based intervention or an experiment. The answer veered towards the latter. Five years on from the launch, how is NICE performing? There have been a large number of outputs as already described, plus the outputs that are less relevant to medicines management – those dealing with interventional procedures. Some of the commentaries on NICE have been described already; additionally the World Health Organization (WHO) reported on the NICE technology appraisal programme in 2003.[42] The WHO report gives an endorsement to the way NICE examines evidence on clinical- and cost-effectiveness. It also states in the executive summary that the 'environment in which NICE functions' – that is, an NHS receiving investment – facilitates achieving NICE objectives – improving quality of care and uptake of technologies. The terms of reference did not include monitoring implementation. A comparison was made between NICE and technology assessments in Australia, Canada, Italy and The Netherlands; NICE was seen as more supportive of novel therapies. WHO did suggest a more explicit approach regarding cost-effectiveness thresholds and provided a number of specific recommendations on process. Reduced transparency when manufacturers' in-confidence material is used was raised as an issue. Overall WHO commented that NICE was having an important influence on NHS decision-making and resource allocation.

This positive message may well have been correct, but there are examples of problems. The implementation of Technology Appraisal 36 (anti-tumour necrosis factors in rheumatoid arthritis), has been cited as a case where variability in delivery has occurred.[43] In spite of the direction to ensure funding (see Department of Health website for 2003 update[44]), this particular therapy was not available as expected over a year later in some areas.[45] A big issue can be the funding for the medicines might be available but the infrastructure costs – clinics, nurses, extra cytotoxic reconstitution costs – may not be received. Further complications can be lack of specialist time and appropriate equipment. These issues should not be overlooked by local health communities in planning and delivering NICE guidance.

Criticism has also been made that health authorities were not monitoring NICE guidance implementation, running the risk that patients are denied treatment.[46] Jones and Strange expressed their concerns, probably reflected in many cancer centres, that the delay between product launch and NICE guidance resulted in greater delays in access to useful therapies.[47] An implication here is that decisions that would have been made in the absence of NICE are delayed to await NICE. The author's view is that even if this is so, it is more than compensated by the access NICE has brought to funds and thus to new therapies. To support the more positive view, Mace and Taylor reported the high perceived take up of the NICE guidance on anticholinesterases for Alzheimer's disease; they surveyed English and Welsh health authority advisers in 2000 and, with a 69% response rate (n = 91), found that nearly 90% believed they were complying with the guidance in their local areas.[48]

In addition to the work led by WHO and the other reports mentioned here, in June 2004, the Department of Health reported their own work undertaken to explore how well NICE appraisals for cancer medicines were being implemented.[49] The Department stated that a number of pharmaceutical companies had expressed concern that the uptake of NICE-approved medicines remained variable. Therefore a review of usage across all English cancer networks was carried out. This was no simple task as the medicines tended to be supplied from hospitals only – collecting such data is difficult because of the lack of a standard reporting mechanism. The key data source was hospital purchasing data sold to IMS Health by hospitals – the report gives a good critique of the weaknesses of such data. Despite this problem, the results emerged to show considerable variation in usage in the period studied (1 July 2003 to 31 December 2003). An example was use of pegylated doxorubicin where there had been no use in one network and over 6 mg per 1000 population in the period in another. The key measure used in the report was a ratio of usage of the 90th percentile to the 10th percentile, a high user compared with a low user but trimming out the extremes. The ratios thus created were always over 2 (where calculable) and in one case as high as 11.61. Although considerable variation was noted, there were some positive messages. The key conclusions were:

- Overall usage of cancer medicines increases once NICE has given a positive appraisal.
- Variation in usage exists and this cannot be explained by 'cross boundary flow' of patients.
- Variation decreases over time.
- Reasons for variation are complex but are thought not to be related to direct funding restrictions, but are more to do with service constraints and different clinical practice.

The last point is interesting, and probably needs further work, but emphasises the importance of local response to NICE guidance. Included in the accompanying papers to the core report were recommendations on how local organisations need to respond; the need for local managerial and clinical leadership to achieve this was emphasised.

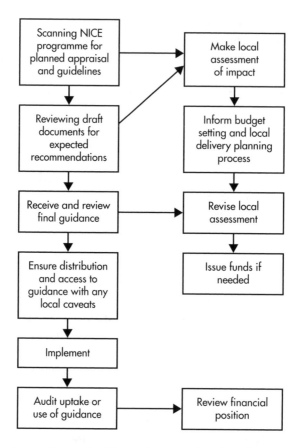

Figure 1.2 Responding to the National Institute for Clinical Excellence.

Further years of planning and delivery rounds are needed and audit or research undertaken over a longer period for a fuller understanding of how health communities are doing in terms of implementing both the technology appraisals and clinical guidelines.

Responding to NICE

How should local organisations respond to NICE? Although the NICE programme goes far beyond medicine use, strategic medicines management does need to include action to respond to NICE. Horizon scanning and budget management are key features in the response; these are discussed in later chapters, as is the implementation of clinical guidelines. Here a brief outline of the possible steps in response to NICE is provided. Figure 1.2 summarises the suggested steps; the NPC issued a detailed practical guide on implementing NICE guidance, which includes a framework and various checklists.[50]

An early view of the NICE programme is required to prepare budget plans, although these can only be guesses until the draft guidance or appraisals are produced. A local impact assessment is necessary. The input of local experts is required to answer questions such as: how many potential patients? Will they all wish to take up therapy? Is the practice identified in the guidance already being followed? Will there be infra-structure costs? Once the NICE documents are final, there needs to be access by those required to implement. Then, assuming affordability has been addressed, there needs to be an assessment of actions required to implement. For negative technology appraisals, action may be required to restrict access; for therapies already in place, a suitable exit strategy is required. A simple enforcement of an existing restriction may need to be continued. Guidance on audit is included in NICE documentation and organisations will need to undertake audit activity to test compli-ance with guidance. For some technology appraisals, documenting uptake of a particular medicine will be easily achieved via prescribing data or, for hospitals without e-prescribing, pharmacy computer systems. However, knowing that a certain number of treatments of a NICE-supported medicine have been supplied does not mean that all patients who should have been offered the treatment have in fact been given that option. With clinical guidelines, a simple analysis of pre-scribing data is unlikely to confirm adherence. Well-designed clinical audit is required to demonstrate this, preferably starting with those patients eligible for treatment, not just those who received it.

Audit of NICE technology appraisal implementation and of clinical guidelines will need to be built into routine audit programmes. Given the volume of documents it is unlikely that all matters will receive regular or full attention. Local organisations will need to prioritise areas where they feel performance may be of concern, or the results of a particular implementation plan need to be tested. How audit pro-grammes are developed is beyond the scope of this book, but use of com-plaints, adverse events and feedback from the patients, carers and users can inform audit prioritisation; such sources are as useful for NICE matters as they are for other issues.

Planning for, assessing the impact of, and implementing and auditing NICE guidance has become a central aspect of strategic medi-cines management for local organisations. The work informs and supports many of the other activities described in this text. Sufficient time and attention need to be given to the NICE programme if organisations are to respond effectively to its recommendations. As described in the Department of Health uptake review of cancer medicines issued in June 2004, 'implementation of recommendations from NICE, as for any service improvement, is not a trivial matter'.[49] Health communities need to take this seriously and ensure that resources to 'make it happen' are there just as much as resources are there to pay for the medicines.

Medicines advice in Scotland

As was mentioned earlier, the work of NICE is aimed at the NHS in England and Wales. Scotland is not excluded from the process but has a well-developed system of its own. NHS Quality Improvement Scotland (NHS QIS) is the body to give advice on standards and to inspect and report on NHS Scotland performance.[51] They advise health boards, who should take action to implement advice. Their website explains that they are involved as a consultee in the development of NICE guidance. They ensure that NICE guidance is issued to healthcare professionals in Scotland at the same time as in England and Wales. However, regarding medicines, there is a body, now under the auspices of NHS QIS, that has the role of issuing guidance on all new medicines: the Scottish Medicines Consortium (SMC), which was set up in 2001. The SMC examines all new medicines, new formulations, and major new indications of established products. Advice is provided in one of three ways: recommended for general use, recommended for restricted use or not recommended. Their annual report for 2003 summarises their work.[52] In 2002, 29 assessments were made; in 2003, 47 full assessments were made, of which 31% the advice 'not recommended' was given. Two examples of advice in the summary are the comments on escitalopram and zoledronic acid. The former was recommended for general use but the guidance noted that the medicine has no clear benefits over the parent molecule or other effective cheaper agents. Zoledronic acid's initial assessment was 'not recommended' owing to lack of data. The second assessment advised restricted use, by oncologists, in cases of multiple myeloma or breast cancer. An independent review of this position confirmed that NHS Scotland should not use zoledronic acid for prevention of skeletal-related events in advanced prostate cancer. SMC notes that where similar medicines are examined, decisions are usually in line with NICE or vice versa.

The 2003 report also included the latest position on the nature of the guidance. Two types of guidance exist, first for unique medicines for specific conditions, second for medicines where alternative therapies exist. On the former, health boards are required to make available all medicines approved by SMC; on the latter, health boards can decide based on local need. This development received the headline 'Scots to cut postcode prescribing' in *The Pharmaceutical Journal*.[53] As with NICE, time is needed to make a judgement on this.

Clinical Resource Efficiency Support Team

The Clinical Resource Efficiency Support Team (CREST) was established in Northern Ireland in 1988. It now comes under the umbrella of the Department of Health, Social Services and Public Safety. Its declared purpose is to balance the need to live within scarce resources while trying to achieve high standards of clinical care.[54] The CREST Drugs Advisory Group was established in September 1997 to lead on issues that relate to the managed introduction of recently licensed drugs that have the potential for major impact in Northern Ireland. The remit of this body is:

- to provide advice to facilitate the managed introduction of recently licensed drugs
- to promote rational, cost-effective and safe prescribing of such drugs
- to promote equity of access to treatment and supply of such drugs for all patients
- to monitor the overall prescribing of such drugs in Northern Ireland.

This seems to go beyond the NICE and SMC remit, moving into performance management or at least monitoring. There have, however, been concerns raised that the failure to automatically apply NICE guidance in Northern Ireland has led to reduced access to medicines. One example, which may seem ironic to those in England with similar worries, was the delays in accessing the anti-tumour necrosis factors for rheumatoid arthritis.[55] Throughout the UK the issues of expectation, evidence and affordability mean that difficult decisions must be made and skilled handling of health resources is required. This is the driving purpose of strategic medicines management.

National Service Frameworks

Another important 'standard setting' programme set out in *The New NHS*, was the National Service Frameworks (NSFs).[13] Their work was further described in *A First Class Service*.[24] This document identified three key roles of NSFs:

- setting national standards and defining service models for a specific service or care group
- putting in place programmes that support implementation
- establishing performance measures with agreed timescales.

Although the guidance is much broader than medicines use, involvement in the delivery of NSFs is seen as vital for primary care trust pharmacy teams.[22] A growing range of NSFs have been developed, some including specific targets relating to medicines. The coronary heart disease standard, published in 2000, includes the very specific target of post-myocardial infarct thrombolysis to be administered within 60 minutes of help being called for the sufferer.[56] This is within one of the twelve standards that cover a range of issues. This target has been a driver for hospitals to reduce door-to-needle times and for ambulance trusts to consider pre-hospital administration of a suitable agent. Such a target does influence availability and choice of product on pragmatic grounds rather than evidence on efficacy alone. Models of care regarding nurse-led service, and paramedic-delivered care, are also raised. In June 2003 it was reported that the percentage of patients administered thrombolysis within 30 minutes of arrival at hospital had risen from 38% in 2000 to 75% in 2003; even if one has doubts about the accuracy of the data from earlier years, this is a sign of significant progress.[57]

An NSF with a very important section on medicines is the one for older people.[58] This NSF has a specific document that deals with medicines, in support of each of the eight main standards: *Medicines and Older People, Implementing Medicines-related Aspects of the NSF for Older People*.[59] Three important milestones were laid down in this document: by 2002 all people over 75 years were expected to have all medicines reviewed annually, and for those having four or more medicines this was to be every six months; one-stop dispensing schemes were to be in place in hospitals along with self-administration schemes; and primary care organisations were to have, by 2004, schemes to ensure that older people got more help from their pharmacists. These are important issues for all organisations, although they relate more to medication management aspects of medicines management than strategic medicines management as has been defined in this text. Nevertheless, organisations taking decisions on the implementation of systems and on specific medicines should ensure that standards set in the NSF are implemented. One important feature of the older person's NSF is that it seeks to eliminate age-related decision making – perhaps ironic when the standard mentioned above has an age target of 75 years – but for drugs committees it would be important to avoid arbitrary cut-off points in guidelines.

The mental health NSF also has a number of medicines-related features.[60] These include the need to find out usage of psychoactive medicines and to have protocols in place. Taylor *et al.* surveyed health authorities in 2001 to see what progress was being made two years on, and found only 6% of returns stated they had completed survey work, although the majority had started work or even completed, a number of protocols.[61]

NSFs on diabetes, for children, cancer and the others all merit attention by those involved in prescribing and medicines use. In addition to the specific standards, milestones and advice each NSF brings, there are more general documents to help implement NSFs. For example, the Department of Health provided a guide to implementation in 2002 that deals with team and organisational aspects of implementation.[62]

For those involved with strategic medicines management, linkage with those leading NSFs locally is important. There should be a review of the NSF and working documents developed locally to check for principles and standards that affect strategic medicines management decisions. It may be that some positive action to change local guidelines or commission guideline work to embed NSF standards is required. Once an NSF is published, strategic medicines management work needs to be informed by its requirements. Organisational aspects of medicines management are considered in the next chapter, but it is worth noting that conflict can result between implementation groups for NSFs and local prescribing committees if there is a failure to develop links and ensure good communications. NSFs are drivers to improve care, including medicines use. Strategic medicines managers need to engage with this process at a local level.

Conclusion

The chapter has dealt with some long-standing influences on local medicines management and the national standard setting NICE, other UK countries' groups and the NSFs. There are other policy drivers and national bodies. The clinical governance agenda and the Healthcare Commission, have been and remain important checks on the way medicines are managed. Developing high-quality systems of decision making is consistent with the general aim of seeking excellence that clinical governance sets. Good medicine use, appropriate access and equity are general principles that apply to strategic medicines management work. The national bodies and standard setting inform and support good medicines use in local, organisations and health communities but they have not taken away the need for local bodies to manage medicines and take decisions on the use of resources. These themes are developed in subsequent chapters.

References

1. Coulter A. Paternalism or partnership? Patients have grown up and there's no going back. *Br Med J* 1999; 319: 719–720.
2. Donaldson L. Expert patients usher in a new era of opportunity for the NHS. *Br Med J* 2003; 326: 1279.
3. Ryan M, Yule B. The way to economic prescribing. *Health Policy* 1993; 25: 25–38.
4. Department of Health. *Statistical Bulletin 2003/12: Prescriptions Dispensed in the Community Statistics 1999–2002, England.* London: DH, 2003.
5. NHS Executive. *Health Service Guideline*, HSG(97)16. London: DH, 1997.
6. Beardon P, Gilchrist M, McKendrick A. *et al.* Primary non-compliance with prescribed medication in primary care. *Br Med J* 1993; 307: 846–848.
7. Freemantle N, Bloor K. Lessons from international experience in controlling pharmaceutical expenditure 1: influencing patients. *Br Med J* 1996; 312: 1469–1471.
8. Schafheutle E. Do high prescription charges undermine compliance? *Pharm J* 2003; 270: 336–337.
9. Walley T. Prescription charges: change overdue. *Br Med J* 1998; 317: 487–488.
10. Scottish Home and Health Department. *Limits to the Range of Products Available under the NHS.* Edinburgh: SHHD, 1985.
11. British Medical Association and the Royal Pharmaceutical Society. *British National Formulary,* 47th edn, London: BMA and RPS, 2004.
12. Yule B, Fordyce I, Bond C, Taylor R. The limited list in general practice: implications for the costs and effectiveness of prescribing. *HERU Discussion Paper No. 1/88.* Aberdeen: University of Aberdeen, 1988.
13. Department of Health. *The New NHS – Modern, Dependable.* London: DH, 1997.
14. Crump B, Panton R, Drummond M *et al.* Transferring the costs of expensive treatments from secondary to primary care. *Br Med J* 1995; 310: 509–512.
15. Rao S. A more creative approach to budget setting? *Primary Care Pharm* 2001; 2: 65–66.
16. Harris C, Scrivener G. Fundholders' prescribing costs: the first five years. *Br Med J* 1996; 313: 1531–1534.
17. Wilson R, Hatcher J, Barton S, Walley T. General practice fundholders' prescribing savings in one region of the UK 1991–1994. *Health Policy* 1997; 42: 29–37.
18. Baines D, Brigham P, Phillips D *et al.* GP fundholding and prescribing in UK general practice: evidence from two rural English Family Health Services Authorities. *Public Health* 1997; 111: 321–325.
19. Ashworth M, Golding S, Shepherd L, Majeed A. Prescribing incentive schemes in two NHS regions: cross sectional survey. *Br Med J* 2002; 324: 1187–1188.
20. Ashworth M, Lea R, Gray H *et al.* The development of prescribing incentive

schemes in primary care. A longitudinal survey. *Br J Gen Pract* 2003; 53: 468–470.

21. Sullivan F. Community: prescribing incentive schemes – more evidence needed on how they work. *Br Med J* 2002; 324: 1187–1188.

22. National Prescribing Centre. *PCT Responsibilities Around Prescribing and Medicines Management.* Liverpool: NPC, 2003.

23. Panton R, Earl-Slater, Grant E. Rising expenditure on medicines – reasons and responses. In Panton R, Chapman S, eds. *Medicines Management.* London: BMJ Publishing Group and Pharmaceutical Press, 1998.

24. Department of Health. *A First Class Service: Quality in the New NHS.* London: DH, 1998.

25. Smith R. NICE: a panacea for the NHS. *Br Med J* 1999; 318: 823–824.

26. National Institute for Clinical Excellence. http://www.nice.org.uk (accessed 8 December 2004).

27. National Institute for Clinical Excellence. *Compilation: Summary of Guidance to the NHS in England and Wales, Issue 7.* London: NICE, 2003.

28. National Institute for Clinical Excellence. *Technology Appraisal No. 55: Guidance on the Use of Paclitaxel in the Treatment of Ovarian Cancer.* London: NICE, 2002.

29. National Institute for Clinical Excellence. *Technology Appraisal No. 77: Zalepon, Zolpidem and Zopiclone for the Short Term Management of Insomnia.* London: NICE, 2004.

30. National Institute for Clinical Excellence. *Technology Appraisal No. 79: New Drugs for Epilepsy in Children.* London: NICE, 2004.

31. National Institute for Clinical Excellence. *Technology Appraisal No. 32: Beta-interferon and glatiramer acetate for multiple sclerosis.* London: NICE, 2002.

32. Kmietowicz Z. News round up: NICE's appraisal procedures attacked. *Br Med J* 2000; 321: 980.

33. Smith R. The failings of NICE. *Br Med J* 2000; 321: 1363–1364.

34. National Institute for Clinical Excellence. *Technology Appraisal No. 15: Guidance on the Use of Zanamivir (Relenza) in the Treatment of Influenza.* London: NICE, 2000.

35. Rawlins M. The failings of NICE, reply from the chairman of NICE [letter]. *Br Med J* 2001; 322: 489.

36. Cookson R, McDaid D, Maynard A. Wrong SIGN, NICE mess: is national guidance distorting allocation of resources. *Br Med J* 2001; 323: 743–745.

37. Dent T, Sadler M. From guidance to practice: why NICE is not enough. *Br Med J* 2002; 324: 842–845.

38. Towse A, Pritchard C, Devlin N. *Cost-Effectiveness Thresholds: Economic and Ethical Issues.* London: King's Fund, OHE, 2002.

39. National Institute for Clinical Excellence. *Inherited Clinical Guideline: Myocardial Infarction Prophylaxis – Drug Treatment, Cardiac Rehabilitation and Dietary Manipulation.* London: NICE, 2001.

40. National Institute for Clinical Excellence. *Clinical Guideline 1: Core Interventions in the Treatment and Management of Schizophrenia in Primary and Secondary Care* London: NICE, 2002.

41. Wailoo A, Roberts J, Brazier J, McCabe C. Efficiency, equity, and NICE clinical guidelines. *Br Med J* 2004; 328: 536–537.

42. World Health Organization. *Technology Appraisal Programme of the*

National Institute of Clinical Excellence. A review by WHO. June–July 2003. Copenhagen: WHO, 2003.

43.   National Institute for Clinical Excellence. *Technology Appraisal No. 36: Entanercept and Infliximab for Rheumatoid Arthritis.* London: NICE, 2002.

44.   Department of Health. National Health Service Act 1977: Further directions to primary care trusts and NHS trusts in England concerning arrangements for the funding of technology appraisal guidance from the National Institute for Clinical Excellence (NICE). http://www.dh.gov.uk/PublicationsAndStatistics/Publications/PublicationsLegislation/PublicationsLegislationArticle/fs/en?CONTENT_ID=4093080&chk=WU9TKZ (accessed 13 December 2004).

45.   BBC News website. http://news.bbc.co.uk/1/hi/health/3126757.stm (accessed 8 December 2004).

46.   Anon. Health Authorities not monitoring compliance with NICE guidance. *Pharm J* 2001; 267: 805.

47.   Jones S, Strange S. Controversy surrounding high-cost drug use in oncology. *Hosp Pharm* 2002; 9: 275–277.

48.   Mace S, Taylor D. Adherence to NICE guidance for the use of anticholinesterases for Alzheimer's disease. *Pharm J* 2000; 269: 680–681.

49.   Department of Health. Variations in usage of cancer drugs approved by NICE. http://www.dh.gov.uk/PublicationsAndStatistics/Publications/PublicationsPolicyAndGuidance/PublicationsPolicyAndGuidanceArticle/fs/en?CONTENT_ID=4083901&chk=vKfY2d (accessed 16 June 2004).

50.   National Prescribing Centre. *Implementing Nice Guidance: a Practical Handbook for Professionals.* Abingdon: Radcliffe Medical Press, 2001.

51.   NHS Quality Improvement Scotland. http://www.nhshealthquality.org (accessed 8 December 2004).

52.   Scottish Medicines Consortium. *Annual Report 2002–2003.* http://www.scottishmedicines.org.uk/updocs/SMC%20ANNUAL%20REPORT.pdf (accessed 8 December 2004).

53.   Anon. Scots to cut postcode prescribing. *Pharm J* 2003; 271: 767.

54.   Clinical Resource Efficiency Support Team. http://www.crestni.org.uk (accessed 8 December 2004).

55.   BBC News website. http://news.bbc.co.uk/1/hi/northern_ireland/2942358.stm (accessed 8 December 2004).

56.   Department of Health. *Coronary Heart Disease: National Service Framework for Coronary Heart Disease: Modern Standards and Service Models.* London: DH, 2000.

57.   NHS Modernisation Agency. *Newsbeat.* Spring/Summer 2003, London: NHS Modernisation Agency, 2003.

58.   Department of Health. *Modern Standards and Service Models: Older People National Service Framework.* London: DH, 2001.

59.   Department of Health. *Medicines and Older People, Implementing Medicines-related Aspects of the NSF for Older People.* London: DH, 2001.

60.   Department of Health. *A National Service Framework for Mental Health, Modern Standards and Service Models.* London: DH, 1999.

61.   Taylor D, Mace S, Young C. Health authority adherence to prescribing related requirements of the NSF for mental health. *Pharm J* 2001; 267: 753–754.

62.   Department of Health. *National Service Frameworks: a Practical Aid to Implementation in Primary Care.* London: DH, 2002.

2

Organisational approaches at a local level

The anonymous cynic, whose words are included in the *Oxford Concise Dictionary of Quotations*, advises us that a committee is a group of the unwilling, chosen from the unfit, to do the unnecessary.[1] This chapter perhaps seeks to convince the reader that a prescribing committee is in fact the dedicated chosen from the able, undertaking difficult but essential tasks – or at least that is what such groups ought to be.

Strategic medicines management comprises a number of activities that have been grouped together in this book. To ensure that these activities are overseen and coordinated at a local level, some sort of organisational structure is required. In the UK and beyond, the drug and therapeutic committee or prescribing committee has been developed to take such a role. This chapter explores the evolution of these committees and their working methods. The impact of the most recent NHS changes will be considered and a model proposed for application in this new environment. There is a considerable literature on these committees' work in Europe, the USA, Australia, Canada and elsewhere. This chapter focuses on the UK picture. Research on effectiveness or impact of prescribing or therapeutic committees is scarce, and in any case difficult to generalise, because the impact depends on the context and functions. Context and functions vary considerably over time and geographically. It is probably very hard to establish what the specific impact of simply having a committee has on medicines use. Indeed it could be argued that seeking information on this is meaningless as it is the tasks overseen or the implementation of decisions that is key, although even studying these more meaningful questions is difficult. Chapter 10 returns to the theme of research.

Titles as well as functions have been quite varied. Unless there is a specific reason for using another title, the term 'drug and therapeutic committee' (DTC) will be used as a tag of convenience to encompass any prescribing, pharmacy and medicines, medicines management or therapeutic committee or group that fulfils a function that is key to strategic medicines management at local level. As encountered in the Introduction, terms tend to vary in their meaning, and as NHS structure has changed, so have committee names – 'area', 'district', 'trust' and so on. Some of these issues will be discussed in a little more detail in the following pages.

The emergence of drug and therapeutic committees

In 1975 a summary of the then current distribution and functions of hospital DTCs was reported by Brown, Barrett and Herxheimer.[2] Their survey across English regions (80% replies, $n = 150$) established that 72% of hospitals had committees of some sort that examined medicines usage, although only 10% reported working on rationalisation of prescribing. Their term was 'hospital pharmacy committee'; they stated that the first was established in 1948 but that most were set up in the late 1960s.

In 1978 the Department of Health and Social Security organised a conference to consider the role of DTCs and then set up a coordinating centre in 1980, based in Southampton. The Professor of Clinical Pharmacology at Southampton University supported by the Principal Pharmacist at the Wessex Drug and Medicines Information Centre undertook a survey from this centre to examine the work going on throughout the UK.[3] They sought information from all health districts in the UK and replies confirmed the existence of 186 DTCs, including 9 in Wales, 18 in southern Scotland and 8 in Northern Ireland. It was fairly clear that the DTCs were a heterogeneous group – for example, size varied from 2 to 23 members.

Although the focus of DTC was the hospital, general practitioners were included in a minority of committees. The most common function was the control of a formulary; second, a role described as the economic use of medicines and, third, safety. It was unusual for a DTC to have executive power – that is, they were not bodies whose decisions had management authority.

Ten years on from the conference, the Department of Health issued a health circular that focused on clinical pharmacy but did stress the importance of DTCs.[4] Similar documents were issued in the other UK countries. The summary of DTC purpose was stated as providing a mechanism for securing the agreement and commitment of clinicians to a rationalised system of medicine usage. The DTC was also to provide an executive group to formulate, implement and monitor the formulary management system aimed at cost-containment. The circular dealt with hospitals but contained important principles relevant to DTCs and strategic medicines management in general. The DTC as a mechanism of gaining 'buy-in' from medical staff is vital. Getting the most from medicines is a multiprofessional activity – of course, involving the patients and public too – but certainly not just a pharmacy responsibility. The idea of an executive group – invested with power to decide and act – is also important. This is not a simple matter and is made more complex with the development of interorganisational DTCs. However, to give advice with no ability to ensure that it is followed, is of little benefit to anyone. As well as laying down these important principles, the health circulars gave a real impetus to DTCs in addition to their important endorsement of clinical pharmacy.

By 1992 DTCs had developed and become the norm. Leach and Leach reported results of their survey of district and chief pharmaceutical officers throughout the UK (returns from 81%, $n = 162$).[5] Of these 57% were organised on a district basis, 19% on a unit basis (this was the term for directly managed hospitals, yet to become trusts) and 21% on a trust basis. Membership varied from 4 to 26. There was a perceptible trend towards accountability at a trust level rather than on a district basis, although the majority remained at district level. Regarding the traditional role of protecting hospital drug budgets irrespective of primary care impact, about 59% stated they considered primary care costs but 63% said the hospital cost was the overriding factor.

NHS structural changes in the early 1990s leading to the provider–purchaser split contributed to further evolution of DTCs. In 1994 Department of Health guidance was issued that emphasised the importance of prescribing in healthcare.[6] The executive letter dealt with the purchasing and prescribing of medicines and the concept of an interorganisational DTC was suggested. The two key objectives stated in the executive letter were ensuring the appropriateness of hospital-led prescribing and the improved management of new medicines into the NHS. The need to have discussions between primary and secondary care was promoted and the development of local arrangements, supported by the contracting process. After this, Leach suggested some of the ways DTCs needed to evolve alongside the NHS changes to ensure that effective dialogue could be established.[7]

Fitzpatrick undertook a survey of English hospital trusts, via directors of pharmacy, in 1994.[8] A 43% response rate ($n = 63$) was achieved, with additional responses from a wider distribution of the same survey to clinical directors. An increase in formation of hospital DTCs was reported with the arrival of trust status, taking the total to 97% of trusts having such a group (among responders). Of the DTCs described, around 5% were set up as district prescribing committees. This suggested a drift away from the 57% arranged in such a way in the 1992 Leach and Leach survey. This may reflect the different methodology or could be seen as a result of the attempt by trusts to show their independence from the primary care community. One role that saw a large increase was the move from 7% of DTCs having a responsibility in requesting funding for medicines pre-trust status, to 20% having such a role when a trust. One conclusion from the work was that additional expert advice on assessing the evidence was needed by DTCs.

Fundholding and greater partnership between primary care practices were developing in this period. Frustration regarding the inequitable access to medicines also grew. One attempt to deal with some of these pressures was the development of a variant DTC, the Midland Therapeutic Review and Advisory Committee (MTRAC). This group aimed to provide a review system to identify the clinical value, safety and suitability of medicines for primary care and to manage the safe introduction of medicines for primary care in that region of England. MTRAC was established in 1995 with GPs as the core decision-making members but supported by public-health doctors, pharmacists, a health economist and other experts. From its start to April 1997, MTRAC reviewed 41 products, of which 16 were new.[9] Clearly this DTC was not the norm and was perhaps a NICE manqué. MTRAC issued three possible rulings:

- recommended for use in primary care
- restricted use in primary care
- not recommended for use in primary care.

The restricted-use category was qualified by three possible conditions: use was considered acceptable if back-up support was available, or if a suitable shared care guideline was produced, or if an individual GP had particular knowledge or skills to enable them to prescribe. The approach was, in essence, to give advice to empower GPs to say no to some of the prescribing shifting taking place from secondary to primary care. The categorisation of medicines adopted by MTRAC has been used in many areas. Typically a traffic light classification is used: red means hospital only, amber is for shared care or restricted use, green is for GP use and GP initiation. Shared care guidelines are discussed in a little more detail in Chapter 7.

It is worth noting another important stream of work that began as early as 1991 in Wessex and at a national level led by the NHS Executive's research and development arm. This could more accurately be described as precursor work to NICE, and involved the development and evaluation committee work and the health technology assessment programme. These were much broader than medicines and it would be misleading to call the groups DTCs, but there are parallels. The Standing Group on Health Technology Assessment at national level was seen as concentrating on a limited range of technologies and taking time to report. The Wessex Evaluation Committee sought to provide rapid evidence-based advice to help healthcare purchasers (now termed commissioners) make purchasing/investment decisions. The approach taken is revisited in the discussion of health economics in Chapter 5. These initiatives were seen as helpful attempts to bring evidence into a difficult area of work, but were subject to criticism – just as NICE has been. Freemantle and Mason reflected on the work evaluation committees had done and what NICE needed to do to improve; they suggested more of the data needed to be available than the evaluation committees usually had (not just published work). They also pointed out that single medicine appraisal was not as helpful as broad class review and they suggested concentrating on what gets marketed rather than scanning the horizon.[10] The last point means that high-quality rapid appraisals must be undertaken at or around product launch. This is quite a challenge and if no time is spent on horizon scanning, even with a positive appraisal there may be no funding for the development.

Following the Labour election victory in 1997 a massive shift in NHS organisation began. The financial flows are mentioned in Chapter 1. Organisational changes followed, with the eventual development of primary care trusts (PCTs) in England and, with the devolved government, new structures in other UK nations. District health authorities and regions were dissolved, leaving strategic health authorities as the overarching performance management organisations. PCTs act as commissioning bodies as well as providing care, whereas the NHS trusts provide acute and specialist care. This process moved in a stepped manner from 1997 to 2003. NHS foundation trusts are in their early days at the time of writing. For medicines management, in addition to budget changes, it meant new communities based around PCT clusters would be the revised landscape of the NHS in England.

At the time the NHS changes began, another DTC development took place. The London New Drugs Group was created. Sharrott reported a key motivator for this DTC was the concern that 'it was not helpful for each health authority to do its own thing'.[11] The group provides advice for London health communities based on evidence and by a consensus of the region's clinical experts. This cross-community

advice, along with MTRAC and development and evaluation committees was endorsed by the NPC document *GP Prescribing Support*.[12]
Published in 1998 it pointed to the 'real advantages in agreeing policy
on certain prescribing issues across a whole geographical area.'

In an article that echoes our anonymous opening quote, Furber
suggested that these DTCs for whole areas were not as beneficial as was
being suggested.[13] The duplication of effort by having organisation and
area-level DTCs, and the redundancy of committees owing to the existence of NICE and other national guidance was pointed out. Although
the reality does not seem to be matched by Furber's concerns, there are
important issues raised and the models for the current NHS environment do need to ensure that effort and skilled time are not wasted.
Duplication in providing appraisals locally, when national documents
exist, ought to be avoidable, and cooperation between DTCs should also
assist this.

In 2000 the NPC undertook a survey of English area prescribing
committees (78% return rate, $n = 77$) to establish the then current
activity.[14] They followed up the survey with focus group meetings. Their
advice was published in a guide to good practice for such DTCs which
included the survey findings.[14] They commented that the vast majority
of health authorities (finally dissolved in 2002) had run a functioning
area DTC since 1995, comprising primary and secondary care representatives. The emerging primary care organisations were also being
represented.

The advice given by the NPC was that the area DTC should not
be a final decision-making group, since that was the role of individual
organisations, but that the DTC advice would need to be taken into
account by those organisations. Local organisations were expected to
have their own DTC and there was also an expectation of two-way
communication between these different groups. The document was a
rich source of advice on terms of reference, membership and relationships. In summary, area DTCs were seen as important advisory bodies
with the role of promoting cost-effective medicine use and supporting
integrated healthcare delivery. Figure 2.1 is adapted from the NPC
document and shows the area DTC recommendation development
process. The NPC acknowledged work done at Bury and Rochdale
Health Authority in preparing this.

A particular aspect of DTC work at an organisational level is the
issue of funding for new medicines. The NPC document suggested
the area DTC could give advice to those taking decisions on priorities –
the individual boards. Southampton reported their work to address this

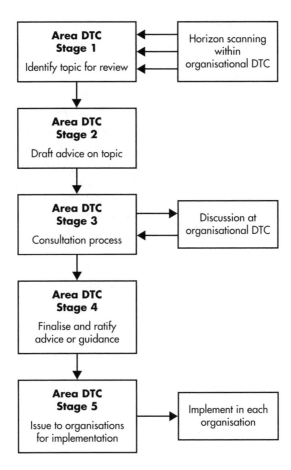

Figure 2.1 National Prescribing Centre advice on drug and therapeutics committee (DTC) recommendation process.

issue in 2000 with further details on their system in 2001.[15,16] At Southampton a DTC subgroup was established in 1998, called the Drug Finance Group, to administer funding of developments on behalf of the trust's DTC. It was a multiprofessional group with primary care membership and it sought to overcome the problem of a DTC wishing to support the introduction of a new medicine but there being no funds to do so.

In 2001, Cantrill and Leese reported the progress being made in English primary care organisations on their new responsibilities with regard to medicines.[17] Based on a 1999 survey, they noted that the vast majority of primary care groups had established their own DTC, described as prescribing subgroups (*n* = 53). Interestingly, whereas the early hospital DTC often included primary care representatives, only two hospital representatives were reported as members of primary care prescribing subgroups.

By late 2001, the Audit Commission's *A Spoonful of Sugar* was published. It was hospital-focused but with comments relevant to the wider DTC agenda.[18] The hospital DTC was seen as key to the effective use of medicines by overseeing controls such as formularies and monitoring usage. The Audit Commission also pointed to the importance of whole-system prescribing arrangements across primary care organisations in England and Wales. The Northamptonshire prescribing project group was commended as a way of improving prescribing and saving money. That DTC dealt with prescribing policies across the primary and secondary care patch and supported some of the initiatives that avoid waste. The issues discussed in Chapter 1 regarding financial flows being unified are addressed in part through the Northamptonshire project group. It does seem that part of the work of current DTCs is to undo some of the work of earlier decades when, to save money on cash-limited budgets, prescribing policy shifts to primary care were encouraged irrespective of what was 'best' for the whole system or for patients.

The move to develop and empower area DTC has continued as the NHS changes have progressed. The Task and Finish Group in Wales supported the move of hospital DTC tasks to primary care organisations ('local health groups' was the term then used in Wales).[19] The model taken up in North Cumbria was reported by Ball and Grainger in 2002.[20] The North Cumbria Medicines Management Group was established in 2001 and took on the responsibilities for all decisions that would affect medicines use in primary care. The two hospital DTCs were merged, but remained in place to consider hospital-only medicines. The local mental health trust retained their own DTC but reported to the area DTC for issues that affected primary care. Local prescribers not implementing recommendations were to be challenged by the medical director and governance officer of the relevant primary care organisation. Similar models are developing around the UK. Burrill reported the work of North Derbyshire's DTC – the Priorities and Clinical Effectiveness Forum.[21] One role included was to take commissioning decisions, thus aligning financial consequences to DTC work.

Throughout the past 30 years of DTC activity, there has been a focus on getting the most from medicines. Organisational changes have been frequent and financial pressures a continuing presence. Not surprisingly, the core functions and responsibilities have changed little during the period, even with the changing environment. The arrival of national bodies that provide advice on medicines has not seen the demise of local DTCs. Indeed one responsibility added to DTC work is the need to ensure implementation of national standards and NICE guidance. As is mentioned in Chapter 1, the expectation in Scotland is that health boards will work through how SMC guidance is implemented for their category II medicines – those where alternative treatments exist.

Before moving on to suggest how DTCs can work in the modern NHS, it is useful to explore the influence of networks and the issue of patient involvement.

The role of networks

The government white paper *The New NHS* identified many changes in organisation of the NHS as already described; it also talked of organising care around a patient's pathway. The concept of the network, already emerged in discussion around cancer services, was being developed. The idea of clinicians, in the broadest sense, working together across a patch to ensure that the best care for patients, lies at the heart of network working. Cancer networks, critical care networks and others have developed. The document laying out principles of cancer care networks emphasised the need for medicines groups – DTCs – that dealt with the specific issues of cancer medicines.[22] It certainly seems wise to support standard regimens across a network patch; supporting entry to trials could be another role, as could exploring dose banding to provide more effective chemotherapy dispensing support. A similar consistency with respect to critical-care medicines, such as activated protein C, would also be logical from a network perspective. A further issue for cancer networks has been the supposedly ring-fenced investment in cancer services. There appeared to be a concern in years of major investment following the 1997 election, that monies aimed at developing cancer services were being lost in trust and PCT deficits. For example, cancer networks wished to be directive in ensuring that funds were used for cancer medicines.

So, how do these networks sit alongside area DTCs, and what are the issues? The members of cancer networks are trusts and PCTs, just as they are for area DTCs. There may be a problem of geography, in that the network patch may not coincide with the prescribing patch. This can lead to boundary issues: one part of the network may have a DTC refusing a development that is supported elsewhere. This problem is slightly reduced by NICE, although not eliminated. There can be a problem of duplication of effort: the cancer DTC reviews a medicine, only for a trust DTC or area DTC to repeat the work. The London cancer drugs groups have tried to produce a consistent multipatch approach to this. The key action must be to establish communication between DTCs and local networks to produce a single-step assessment process that has credibility with all parties. Area DTCs have busy agendas, so receiving advice from a network supported by critically appraised evidence should be welcomed. There is no one right way to do this, but here the pattern of a prescribing patch DTC being the overarching guidance issuing body is suggested as the preferred model.

The role of the patient and the public

The George and Hands survey of DTCs in 1980 recorded consultant, pharmacist, nurse, administrator, junior doctor and GP membership, but no general public or patient members were reported.[3] In 1997, Fitzpatrick reported the position 14 years on.[8] No lay, general public or patient members were mentioned. MTRAC (set up in 1995) included a medical ethicist, described as able to present the patient perspective if the evidence is ambivalent.[9] This was an interesting approach – perhaps now quite patronising – but comparatively progressive based on Fitzpatrick's findings.

The NPC practice guide for DTC did not include patient membership within its core or extended lists of suggested membership but, importantly, a community health council representative or non-executive director was proposed.[14] The two roles were seen as alternatives, although clearly a non-executive director of an NHS body would be perceived as less independent than a member of the community health council.

The NHS Plan, published in July 2000, announced significant changes in the way patients would be involved with their own care and how public involvement with the NHS would be developed.[23] The opening paragraph of Chapter 10 states: 'Patients must have more say in their own treatment and more influence over the way the NHS works.' The patient advocacy and liaison services, to be developed throughout the NHS, were announced, developing the expert patient was supported and its extension included. In the context of the DTC, the key discussion in the plan was around involving patients and 'citizens' at various levels of NHS and regulatory bodies – having patients and the public shape services. With such a move in the NHS at large it would seem neglectful for DTCs to be bastions of professionals only, even if choosing and involving patients is difficult.

In 2001, a discussion document seeking to further develop the involvement of patients was produced.[24] The range of ideas raised in *The NHS Plan* was taken forward. An emphasis on involving patients in significant service changes was made. Further developments, through to the setting up of the Commission for Patient and Public Involvement in Health and the issue of details on the arrangements for patient and public involvement in 2003 have taken place.[25] The arrangements of membership and patient/public involvement in NHS foundation trusts also makes the process of working with the public a reality.

As well as the general documents supporting a patient-centred NHS, the pharmacy-focused plan also sought a greater emphasis on the patient.[26] Watson pointed out some of the ways this can happen at an individual level and for service developments, although she also noted the difficulty of trying to involve patients in meetings where other members are just not used to such inclusion.[27]

The use of local support groups for specific conditions may be a way of consulting on local guidelines and decisions; drawing representatives from patient bodies may be a way of strengthening DTCs. However it is done, it is clear that the move in the NHS is towards including those affected by decisions in the making of decisions. Strategic medicines management needs to embrace this move.

A model for drug and therapeutic committees in the modern NHS

The brief history of DTCs in the NHS identified changes as the environment changed. No one model of structure, function and relationships was ever overwhelmingly dominant and it would be wrong to suggest there is only one right way to organise a DTC. The remainder of the chapter focuses on the features and functions of DTCs in an NHS where NICE, SMC and CREST issue guidance and where, in England, primary care trusts are commissioning bodies. The issues to be discussed are the size and shape of the area covered, the organisational structures of the DTCs, the functions, membership and working relationships of the various DTCs in a patch and how performance might be monitored.

The drug and therapeutic committee's community

When district health authorities were the norm, there was, perhaps, a natural community to cooperate over prescribing matters. Health boards and health groups in Scotland and Wales are possibly still these natural communities. However for England, a single PCT is unlikely to form such an entity. Most district general hospitals will have important commissioning relationships with more than one PCT. Teaching and specialist trusts will have relationships with very large numbers of PCTs. The area DTC arrangements need to be arranged in a way that reflects these new health communities. The examples mentioned earlier, North Cumbria and Derbyshire, attempt to do this. Their area DTCs were different but followed similar patterns. Box 2.1 gives the member organisation structures along with that from the author's own locality. With these revised arrangements in place, perhaps the area DTC needs to be renamed the health community DTC, or even a prescribing patch DTC, to reflect the very real but less formal nature of the joint working.

Another option for an area DTC would be to amalgamate across a larger area – the strategic health authority, perhaps – or at a county level. This may have the advantage of being a well-defined area and may possibly reduce the need for duplication. This level of working has successful examples, MTRAC and the London new drugs group being two. However, if a key principle of DTC work is to ensure the engagement of clinicians to deliver good medicines use, it may be a step too far for some communities. Multi-county DTCs, covering very large populations, may develop for some strategic health authorities, but it

---

Box 2.1 Examples of new area drug and therapeutic committee (DTC) arrangements.

North Cumbria Medicines Management Group

- Three primary care trusts
- Two acute trusts
- Reports from the mental health trust also received

North Derbyshire

- Three primary care trusts
- An acute trust
- A mental health trust

Winchester and Southampton

- Four primary care trusts
- An acute teaching trust
- An acute trust
- A mental health trust

would not be surprising to see local DTCs as an extra layer between it and individual organisational DTCs.

Prescribing patch DTCs, including more than one NHS trust and a group of PCTs, is therefore the suggested approach. This is not without problems. Although there have to be boundaries somewhere, trusts – especially teaching and specialised trusts – will almost certainly provide care for patients beyond their prescribing patch borders. Cancer networks, local authorities, deaneries and specialist commissioning arrangements may well be based on different geographical areas. Arrangements will just not be tidy. Exchange of information, agreeing to derogate decisions to other groups at times and sharing critical appraisal can help smooth out some of these issues. It is very unlikely that teaching trusts or mental health trusts would accept, or could cope with, four or five different prescribing guidelines or policies related to the patient's postcode, although of course patients have had to tolerate different levels of access to medicines dependent on where they live.

Figure 2.2 suggests how these intra- and interpatch relationships could begin to work. As well as the area DTC, there remains a role for PCT prescribing or medicines management groups and for DTCs in NHS trusts. The different functions of these organisational groups will be explored shortly, but they remain the bodies responsible to the boards within each organisation. Accountability of the area DTC is slightly more difficult. If, as has been suggested, the DTC should be at prescribing patch level, not strategic health authority level, then there is no obvious body to which the DTC should be accountable. If the area DTC were to be on a strategic health authority basis, there would still be an issue as managing a DTC directly would not fit with the key role of these organisations. In both cases it may be best to use a confederation-like approach. A joint meeting of leads from PCT executive committees and the executive groups of trusts locally may be a suitable body to oversee the area DTC. Certainly the commitment of individual organisations' executives and boards to the arrangements of DTC is required if they are to be effective.

Drug and therapeutic committee functions

If the suggested structure is accepted, that is, an area DTC that covers a health community supported by individual organisational DTCs, what are the functions of the different bodies? Their overarching purpose is to ensure that medicines management, and in particular strategic medicines management, is of a high standard. But which committee should

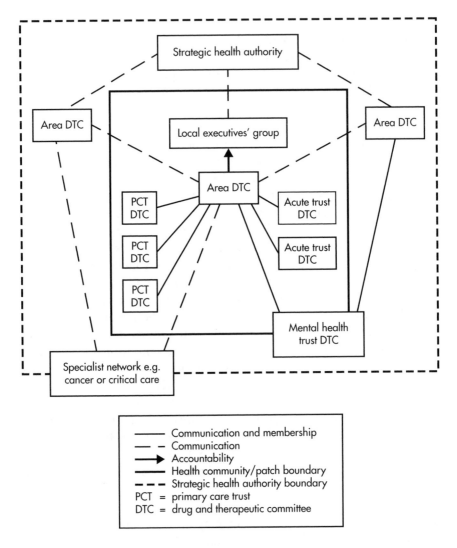

Figure 2.2 Arrangements for drug and therapeutics committees in a health community.

do what? The logical approach is to identify the tasks, then decide which DTC is best placed to do each, taking into account efficient use of resources and the way accountability works.

The following tasks, perhaps with some overlap, describe what needs to be done:

- ensuring that national guidance is available, funded and implemented
- giving local advice and tailoring of national guidance if required

- giving guidance on the use of medicines while national guidance is awaited
- giving guidance on the availability and use of medicines not dealt with by national guidance
- developing formularies or limited lists to control access to medicines
- managing the issues related to the prescribing of complex medicines where primary care prescribing is beneficial but problematic
- monitoring prescribing to ensure that it is evidence-based, cost-effective and affordable
- dealing with unusual cases that fall outside guidance
- dealing with prescribing performance that falls short of expected standards
- monitoring and overseeing expenditure on medicines, in support of budget holders
- dealing with issues of policy related to prescribing at the interface – discharges, one-stop dispensing in secondary care
- dealing with prescribing policy and practice for outpatient services.

These 12 areas of activity fall into the general description of strategic medicines management but other tasks also need to be addressed: patient group directions, extending prescribing responsibility, design of hospital prescribing charts, adverse event reporting, purchasing policies related to medicines, safety-related matters including error monitoring, and induction and training regarding medicines management. If the model of an area DTC is accepted, how would the 12 main functions be distributed, particularly if duplication is to be avoided? Table 2.1 attempts to map them out. This is not a definitive description of a local community's arrangements, as there will be various arrangements and environmental factors. However, the idea of a single-stage evidence review and consistent implementation of advice or guidance is vital for effective DTC working.

The following chapters deal with developing a formulary, horizon scanning and controlled access, guidelines and budgets. DTCs have a key role in ensuring that these activities are in place and work well across organisations. There are two important areas of choice for the model of DTC suggested here. The major role for issuing guidance on medicines not covered by national documents is placed with the area DTC. Should the area DTC be concerned with items only used in secondary care? Should any DTC be concerned about even minor decisions of little clinical or financial consequence? The first question relates to anaesthetic agents and medicines used on critical care, for example. The need to make choices and issue guidance on these agents will not affect general practitioner prescribing, but they may well consume significant resources within the health community. A single evidence review process could include these medicines and an area

Table 2.1 Functions of drug and therapeutic committees (DTCs)

Function	Area DTCs	Organisational DTCs
National guidance		
made available	Minor role	Major role
funded	Advising commissioning process	Advising commissioning process
implemented	Minor role	Major role
Advising on implementation of national guidance	Major role	Minor role but lead implementation
Providing guidance while national guidance awaited	Major role	Minor role but lead implementation
Giving guidance where no national guidance exists	Major role	Minor role but lead implementation
Agreeing formulary or limited list	Major role	Minor role but lead implementation
Managing issues related to complex medicines	Major role	Minor role but lead implementation
Ensuring prescribing is cost-effective and evidence-based	Minor or overseeing role	Major role
Dealing with individual cases where guidance is not seen as applicable	Minor role	Major role
Dealing with poor prescribing performance	Little or no role	Advisory role to management of relevant area
Monitoring expenditure and ensuring prescribing is affordable	Minor or overseeing role but decisions taken in the light of affordability	Major role
Dealing with policy at the interface, e.g. discharge medicines	Major role	Implementing guidance
Ensuring prescribing policies are in place, e.g. for outpatients	Overseeing and role in ensuring consistency	Implementing guidance

prescribing committee could be helpful in prioritising local resource use. Moving the decision making from trust DTC to area DTC may give concern to both parties – secondary care feeling they are losing control, primary care feeling they are dealing with matters outside their experience – but, if done well, this approach could provide a robust, whole-health, community-supported medicines management system.

The second of the questions relates to minor decisions. There will be many competing needs for critical appraisal and DTC time. Some decisions – which topical steroid, whether to use a new, modified-release version of a product in secondary care – may have little consequence, and perhaps scanty evidence, but could take up DTC time. Area DTCs could set a limit on what gets considered, for example, only items likely to have an impact above a set financial figure. Another approach would be to allow a subgroup or even a full DTC to decide how these matters will be handled, delegating some to organisational DTCs or leaving decisions to individual prescribers.

These two issues, as with the detail of structures, need to suit local circumstances. What counts is that there is a system that works, making decisions in good time and supporting prescribers with evidence-based guidance. The model here is of area DTCs issuing guidance or decisions, which the organisational DTCs ensure are implemented, perhaps having some decisions delegated to them. Other models with a slightly different balance may also work.

Membership

Various patterns of membership of DTC have been suggested and used over the years. The key is to have a multiprofessional group with credibility and the skills required to undertake the functions. The exact details will depend on the structures, but for this section the pattern described above and illustrated in Figure 2.2 will be assumed. For the area DTC, each organisation should be represented, perhaps by their prescribing lead or senior clinician and by their lead or chief pharmacist. This brings organisational buy-in and a mix of experience and viewpoint. Commissioning and or financial representation from the local health community would aid communication and add credibility to the DTC decisions. Public health perspective, critical appraisal skills, communication skills and an ability to use health economic data will all add to the strength of the DTC. Executive representation from one or more organisations may also lend it credibility, although primarily the DTC is a clinically focused group, trying to ensure best use of medicines.

The voice of the patient or public needs to be heard, preferably through the input of one or two members, supported so they can effectively contribute to the debate. This is an area for development and, perhaps, research to find an effective model. Nursing, community pharmacist and other healthcare professional views may also help the committee achieve a balanced approach. Local medical committee views on shared care and other matters will also need consideration.

This rather long list will need to be managed carefully to avoid an unworkable arrangement. Numbers growing beyond 14–18 members begin to be difficult to chair, and it is difficult for members to feel they can participate effectively. Clearly, chairing such meetings is a skilled task and requires careful planning. Good secretarial support, with rapid communication of key decisions, is vital. It is important that member organisations send representatives empowered to contribute; it is no good the area DTC agreeing a shared care guideline or restriction of a medicine, if these will not be supported within local organisations.

Organisational DTCs also need to be representative of the range of views in the organisation, multiprofessional and informed by general management and finance. Cross-sector input may not be so important in the model described here – organisational DTCs being more the in-house implementers of area DTC guidance – but if more decisions are taken at local DTC level, then cross-sector input is essential. Risk management could be a feature of trust and primary care trust DTCs, in which case the relevant risk leads need to be present. Patient or public input is again important; a patient's view on a patient group direction could be very helpful. For foundation NHS trusts, the membership council could be a source of such individuals.

Monitoring impact

Chapter 9 discusses performance management, but it is worth mentioning a few aspects of DTC impact here. There are some key questions that summarise how DTCs could be monitored:

- Do the arrangements work? For example, do members attend? How are the arrangements viewed in the local health community?
- Are the important issues addressed?
- Are the decisions made and guidance issued credible locally? Are decisions peer reviewed?
- Is guidance issued in a timely manner – for example, are there long delays in access to medicines or long periods of uncertainty before restrictions are placed?

- Are decisions and guidance communicated to the appropriate people?
- Are the decisions and guidance implemented? For example are shared care guidelines followed? Are medicines used when the DTC decides they ought not to be? What non-formulary prescribing is there?

Regular review of these issues by local organisations and by the DTC will allow a view of performance to be established. Action to improve performance may be needed, including changing structures. The key objective of good medicines usage should be remembered and the work of DTC tested against this.

Conclusion

DTCs have developed and changed over the years. Future change in the NHS will inevitably lead to changes in structure and function of these groups. Where DTCs work well, strategic medicines management should have a group that oversees and supports the various elements. The exact detail and organisational arrangements are probably less important than the performance. Words that echo the 1988 health circulars are key – DTCs should be groups that ensure that clinicians are committed to systems that assist the rational use of medicines at a local level. The arrival of national guidance has not reduced the importance of this role.

References

1. Anon. In Knowles E, ed. *Oxford Concise Dictionary of Quotations*, 4th edn. Oxford: Oxford University Press, 2001.
2. Brown A, Barrett C, Herxheimer A. Hospital pharmacy committees in England: their structure, function and development. *Br Med J* 1975; 1: 323–326.
3. George C, Hands D. Drug and therapeutic committees and information pharmacy services: the United Kingdom. *World Dev* 1983; 11: 229–236.
4. Department of Health. *The Way Forward for Hospital Pharmaceutical Services* HC 88(54). London: DH, 1988. Also WHC 88(66) (Wales) 1988 and 1988 (GEN) 32 for Scotland 1988.
5. Leach S, Leach R. Drug and therapeutic committees in the UK in 1992. *Pharm J* 1994; 253: 61–63.
6. Department of Health. *Executive letter EL(94)72: Purchasing and Prescribing*. London: DH, 1994.
7. Leach R. Why drug and therapeutic committees are set for further change. *Hosp Pharm Pract* 1994; 4: 365.
8. Fitzpatrick R. Is there a place for drug and therapeutic committees in the new NHS? *Eur Hosp Pharm* 1997; 3: 143–147.

9. Blenkinsopp A, Clark W, Purves I, Fisher M. Getting research into practice. In Panton R, Chapman S, eds. *Medicines Management*. London: BMJ Publishing Group and Pharmaceutical Press, 1998: 133–153.

10. Freemantle N, Mason J. Not playing with a full DEC: why development and evaluation committee methods for appraising new drugs may be inadequate. *Br Med J* 1999; 318: 1480–1482.

11. Anon. Managing the entry of expensive new drugs. *Pharm J* 2000; 265: 496–497.

12. National Prescribing Centre and NHS Executive. *GP Prescribing Support: a Resource Document and Guide for the New NHS*. London: NPC and NHSE, 1998.

13. Furber T. If in doubt, form a committee. *Pharm J* 1998; 261: 901–902.

14. National Prescribing Centre. *Area Prescribing Committees – Monitoring Effectiveness in the Modern NHS, a Guide to Good Practice*. Liverpool: NPC, 2000.

15. Stephens M, Tomlin M, Mitchell R. Managing medicines: the optimising drug value approach. *Hosp Pharm* 2000; 7: 256–259.

16. Stephens M. Economic analyses to assist drug entry decision making. *Pharm Manage* 2001; 17: 36–40.

17. Cantrill J, Leese B. An exploration of the potential impact of primary care groups on pharmaceutical practice. *Pharm J* 2001; 266: 857–859.

18. Audit Commission. *A Spoonful of Sugar: Medicines Management in NHS Hospitals*. London: Audit Commission, 2001.

19. National Assembly for Wales. *Report of the Task and Finish Group on Prescribing*. Cardiff: National Assembly for Wales, 2000.

20. Ball K, Grainger I. Evolution of medicines management across primary and secondary care. *Med Manage* 2002; 1: 5–6.

21. Burrill P. Area prescribing committees – what is their role in the new NHS. *Pharm J* 2003; 270: 409.

22. NHS Executive. *Manual of Cancer Services*. London: NHSE, 2000.

23. Department of Health, Chapter 10. *The NHS Plan: a Plan for Investment, a Plan for Reform*. Norwich: The Stationery Office, 2000.

24. Department of Health. *Involving Patients and the Public in Healthcare: a Discussion Document*. London: DH, 2001.

25. Department of Health. Strengthening accountability – involving patients and the public: practice guidance. http://www.dh.gov.uk/PublicationsAndStatistics/Publications/PublicationsPolicyAndGuidance/PublicationsPolicyAndGuidanceArticle/fs/en?CONTENT_ID=4074289&chk=2mwdZZ (accessed 15 December 2004).

26. Department of Health. *Pharmacy in the Future*. London: DH, 2000.

27. Watson C. How concordance and patient empowerment challenge pharmacy. *Pharm J* 2003; 271: 494.

3

Formularies

Formularies dealing with medicines have been in use for many years. Just as the phrase 'medicines management' itself, the word 'formulary' conveys various meanings. Three different usages can be identified: a list of formulas, a restrictive list of medicines and a comprehensive list of medicines. *Butterworths Medical Dictionary* defines 'formulary' as a published list of formulas in general medical use – this in line with the more usual 'ordinary' dictionary term.[1] Although details of formulas are occasionally referred to in healthcare practice, the second and third usages are more common, particularly in the context of medicines management. An example from the not-too-distant past illustrates the restrictive approach: the *National War Formulary* of 1941 states in its preface: 'In preparing the Formulary the aim . . . has been to provide a selection of medicines sufficient in range to meet the ordinary requirements of therapeutics . . . and to eliminate non-essential drugs.'[2] Of course, at such times resources were scarce and 'strictest economy in prescribing' was essential. However, the principles often used in preparing formularies for current organisations are there: list the essential medicines; remove the less useful. The more inclusive approach is taken in the *British National Formulary*, which includes 'drugs that are generally prescribed in the UK', although within the text those that are 'less suitable for prescribing' are identified.[3]

This chapter concentrates on formularies developed at organisational or health community level, where there is an assumption that items not included will have restrictions placed on their use. There is a brief review of how such documents have developed in the NHS, evidence of what is currently in place and evidence of the impact they have. Cost and safety aspects of formulary use will be considered. The impact of electronic prescribing with decision support on formulary management is considered and the chapter ends with suggested options for the place formularies have in the future of medicines management.

Formularies emerge

An early example of a hospital formulary system that fits in with the restrictive approach is the Westminster Hospital Formulary. Baker *et al.*

report that their key motivation for establishing this, in 1970, was to help control expenditure by limiting the choice of products available.[4] They consulted all senior medical staff on the proposed list but found this a rather cumbersome approach and eight years later it was revised. Other hospitals began to build their own formulary systems, often motivated by financial pressures. Middlebrook summarised the progress on formularies during the 1970s, noting that by 1979 around 30% of the small number of hospitals surveyed across the UK had formularies in place.[5] This was slightly more than the numbers that can be extrapolated from the 1975 report, where only 14 hospital 'pharmacy' committees across England, of the 150 hospital responses, stated that their work included 'rationalisation of prescribing', although specific information on formularies was not reported.[6]

These initial steps in secondary care were also seen in general practice; in 1981 personal formularies were suggested as a way to improve prescribing in primary care.[7] From the early 1980s examples of formularies used by all partners rather than just individuals began to appear and were mentioned in the literature. In 1985, Green described the work in Runcorn supported by Mersey Regional Research Committee from 1981; Grant *et al.* reported work undertaken in Newcastle to develop a formulary that covered 90% of patients' needs and sought to improve the quality of prescribing.[8,9] Later in the 1980s the *Lothian Formulary* and the *Practice Formulary* in Northern Ireland were developed, each aimed at providing a reduced list of medicines for regular use, and so contained fewer than 10% of the items listed in the *British National Formulary*.[3,10,11]

By 1986 *The Nuffield Report* into pharmacy was able to cite drug and therapeutic committees in hospitals as important bodies for interprofessional work and the source of formulary development 'in a number of cases'.[12] By 1989 the *Drug and Therapeutics Bulletin* pointed to around half of NHS organisations having formularies with 'some practices' having their own.[13] Their comments were, in part, based on work undertaken by Ridley of Social Audit, who surveyed district health authorities' publishing findings in 1986.[14] Commenting on Ridley's work, Petrie and Scott noted that there were still blocks to formulary development, vigorous defence of clinical freedom being one of significance.[15] However, during 1988, production of formularies in hospitals received a boost with the issue of the various *Way Forward* health circulars that supported their use, alongside an endorsement of clinical pharmacy services and drug and therapeutic committees.[16] An 'allocation of pharmacists to assist in the development and maintenance of a formulary' to help contain expenditure on medicines was a required action.

Work to implement formulary systems throughout UK hospitals was supported by further documents and statements.[17–19] Thus, by 1993, Joshi *et al.* were able to report 91% of responding hospitals as having formularies in place.[20] The survey covered all UK acute general hospitals with more than 500 beds; an 89% response rate was achieved from the 74 questionnaires issued. They used Ridley's definition of formulary: any list of selected drugs from which hospital doctors are encouraged or required to prescribe.[14] They asked when the formularies had been introduced and noted a few early implementers (six in the 1970s) but that the majority had introduced them during the 1980s (70% of those who had one in place). With such levels of uptake, not surprisingly, the focus began to move from 'Is there a formulary?' to 'What is the formulary system and is it working in a joined-up way?' This sophistication will be revisited, but with the consolidation of formularies in secondary care, what was happening in general practice?

A Prescription for Improvement was published in 1994.[21] It contained a revealing definition of a formulary: 'list of selected drugs, sometimes accompanied by guidance and protocols for their use, compiled by most hospitals, a few districts or FHSAs [family health service authorities], some GP practices, and also some published by also [*sic*] academic departments (Belfast, Newcastle, Lothian, etc).' In the document, the Audit Commission put forward, as examples of good practice, those that had developed formularies. Just as in the 1980s hospitals had pursued the formulary path, the 1990s saw practices and primary care organisations taking on their development.

In 1998, the National Prescribing Centre, with the NHS Executive, produced *GP Prescribing Support: a Resource Document and Guide for the New NHS*.[22] As well as giving several examples of primary care formularies, it pointed out the importance of having a formulary system. It also stressed the benefits of the process of maintaining the formulary, as well as the advantage GPs have in using a formulary because of their computer systems.

Following the publication of *The New NHS: Modern, Dependable* in 1997, significant changes took place in the organisation of primary care in England, culminating in all primary care organisations having become primary care trusts (PCTs) by April 2002.[23,24] These changes meant that general practices were brought together into organisations where both provision of healthcare and commissioning of healthcare took place. Pharmacy teams working at practice and organisational levels could support the development of formularies and look towards joint working with their provider hospitals. This becomes particularly important in the light of the financial changes running alongside the organisational ones, as Chapter 1 describes. Joint formularies were predicted, began to be written up in the literature and stated as good practice.[25–29] The 2003 medicines management in NHS trusts framework in England highlighted the need for therapeutic consistency across primary and secondary care.[30] It can be noted that in Scotland this development had been proposed earlier, with the 1993 Scottish Office Circular.[31]

Thus in a period of around 30 years, an innovation – the formulary that states the medicines that are the preferred first choice – had spread, become accepted practice and had been adapted to suit the needs of a changed NHS. Readers can judge if this was rather laboured progress or the inevitable rate of development for an intervention that has a variety of styles and structures.

What kind of formulary?

This chapter opens with comments regarding different meanings of the term 'formulary'. An approach settled on was a listing of medicines for use, where restrictions applied to items not on the list. However, this is rather vague and, although in describing the emergence of formularies, content has had mention, the design of formularies merits further discussion. Certainly this is so if the question 'Do formularies work?' is to be addressed.

Four key dimensions can be applied to formularies to describe their nature. Table 3.1 details a way of describing these. In summary they are: character, coverage, compulsion and community. The character or style of a formulary can be a simple list or a set of guidelines detailing how the medicines are to be used. For hospitals, the simple list is not considered adequate, with links to diagnosis being proposed by the Audit Commission and use of guidelines expected in the medicines management framework.[30,32] The range of possible styles is best viewed as a continuum: at the simple end, a list of drugs available in whatever preparation is required, through sophistications where medicines are listed, sometimes with 'limits' on use, to a comprehensive document where algorithms linked to clinical situations are developed for all medicines available.

The detail added, which moves the formulary beyond a simple list, may be related to preparations available or circumstances in which prescribing may be considered 'outside the formulary'. Thus a formulary

Table 3.1 Formulary designs

Feature	Approach or style taken		
Character	Simple list	List with sophistications	Collation of guidelines
Coverage	Selected therapeutic areas		Comprehensive
Compulsion	Preferred or suggested list	Some compulsion or control or compulsion for some groups	Adherence required of all
Community	Local application for single organisational needs	Local application with consultation or consideration of partners	Joint primary and secondary document for a whole 'patch'

may include an oral medicine, but not in its modified release form, or the document may indicate which medicine is first line and which second line for a particular indication. This approach falls short of a comprehensive set of guidelines but, at face value, appears more helpful to the prescriber than a simple listing. Joshi *et al.* described two-thirds of the hospital formularies they identified in their early 1990s study as being more than just simple lists, although the addition of dosage forms was the most common sophistication (in 80%) and the addition of indications the next most common (in 60%).[20] Box 3.1 provides an example of a formulary entry that provides a reasonable level of information without being a true guideline.

The second of the Cs – coverage – deals with the question: 'Does the formulary attempt to deal with all or only a limited range of therapeutic areas?' Certainly to attempt to cover every possible therapeutic intervention in a large multispeciality tertiary centre at first draft of a formulary would be an awesome task. To use an example from the author's own patch, antibiotics were addressed first, in 1978, before a full listing of all *British National Formulary* sections was produced in 1985.[33,34] This stepped approach can allow some benefits to be gained before the total investment to develop a document is complete. The general practice project in Newcastle sought to cover 90% of treatment needs with their first formulary, deliberately excluding emergency- and hospital-initiated medicines.[9] The stepped approach could also be used in converting lists into guidance and hospital or general practice formularies into joint documents. The *Wessex Formulist* attempted this, with

---

Box 3.1 A hospital formulary extract. (The examples are illustrative and do not indicate support for the selected medicines over other agents in these classes.)

Section 2.5.5 Drugs affecting the renin–angiotensin system

2.5.5.1 Angiotensin-converting enzyme inhibitors

Please note not to be used as first line for hypertension
Caution: first dose hypotension, renal disease, see BNF for further details.
Enalapril
Lisinopril
Ramipril

2.5.5.2 Angiotensin II receptor antagonists

Please note only for use where an ACE inhibitor has been tried but not tolerated
Losartan
Candesartan
Irbesartan *NB only available to elderly care and endocrinology team*

---

guidance on upper gastrointestinal tract disease, depression, migraine, intermittent claudication, benign prostatic hypertrophy and typhoid vaccination – quite an eclectic set.[35]

The level of compulsion that a formulary brings is a more emotive topic than whether all *British National Formulary* chapters are covered. Practice has varied over the years and between organisations. Ridley reported that, within some hospitals, formularies included entries which were available only to specialists, whereas other styles listed medicines available to all prescribers.[14] Joshi *et al.* found that about half the hospitals surveyed made formulary adherence compulsory for junior doctors but voluntary for consultants.[20] This was a practice they described as questionable, such use only bringing partial control, lessening any impact of the document.

A common theme is that formularies work on the basis that most patient needs can be met for most of the time. Typically, even without compulsion, prescribing within the formulary is reported to be at levels of around 90%. Access to medicines not listed may be reduced even if 'prohibition' is not used. Thus, in hospital, the pharmacy may not stock non-formulary medicines, resulting in a delayed availability of such products. An extra step or barrier may be introduced for non-formulary or 'second-line' formulary medicines. In hospital practice this may mean requiring a consultant countersignature, or a conversation with the clinical pharmacist, or confirmation of need by a microbiologist. In a general practice or a hospital where electronic prescribing is in place, a non-formulary choice may need extra work – questions to be answered or full typing rather than a prompted regimen.

For whom is the formulary intended is the final C – community. A range of different documents have been described in this chapter already: a single hospital formulary, one for a single general practice, and a whole-health community formulary. It would seem attractive to have a document to which all can contribute and all can use, rather than different or conflicting documents in a health community. Table 3.1 identifies three approaches: an organisation developing a formulary in isolation, an organisation producing their own formulary but seeking acceptance and support from others in the health community, and a truly joint formulary. In the early days, hospital formularies concentrated on hospital prescribing, as mentioned previously. In fact some prescribing switches actually compromised primary care medicine use. Loss leading by pharmaceutical companies, where very large discounts were provided to hospitals to promote one brand, encouraged use of particular nitrates or combination products. Later, the impact of formulary decisions on primary care began to be considered, then began to influence formularies. Such involvement or influence could exist without the move to a joint document – a document used in both sectors of care. However, as general practice and PCT formularies become more common, having different medicines in a particular class can only lead to confusion – perhaps conflict. Thus if a certain statin is chosen as first line for most patients in a PCT, for the local district general to choose another would result in either continual switching or non-adherence in both places. How important this is depends on our view of formularies. The evidence of their impact is assessed later, but at face value inefficiencies seem likely. If a local health community does not have a joint formulary, perhaps some practices working with no agreed formulary and others with different lists, a one step move to a comprehensive single document may be unrealistic. It may take considerable effort to gain agreement on all therapeutic areas across all practices. Even with genuine commitment, there is a large amount of work required. Concentrating on key therapeutic areas, new introductions and secondary care-led medicines, may be the wisest approach. Then over a period of time a document can emerge, with an increasing level of coverage as each step is taken.

Do formularies work?

The Audit Commission is very clear that, for hospitals, establishing a formulary is a crucial part of effective medicines management – 'the cornerstone' is how it is described.[32] They argue that problems will result in the absence of formulary systems: more errors, higher costs, supply difficulties and greater waste. Intuitively, such consequences appear likely, but what is the evidence base for the statements? What evidence is there that formularies work? Here, the aspects of quality of prescribing and cost will be addressed – the intended outcomes of formulary systems – but the issue of adherence or compliance will be considered first – more to do with process. This is important in considering the evidence of impact, since having a formulary that is ignored by all is unlikely to have an impact on quality or on costs, although it would be wrong to assume that a formulary with low adherence, 50% for example, is not improving these aspects of prescribing. To work through an example, a multipartner general practice may introduce a formulary with just one statin, to permit cost-effective prescribing and ensure that all patients have the right dose regimen; after 18 months, 50% of prescribing may be of the chosen statin, delivering definite savings and straightforward regimens compared with a spread of prescribing across five or six statins previously used.

The early work on a hospital formulary by Baker *et al.* found formulary adherence difficult to achieve with their first attempt.[4] Their initial model was too cumbersome – all consultants were asked to approve the list and any subsequent change. However, they found by having an 'executive group' who sought expert comments from relevant specialists, as needed, and investing pharmacist time, they achieved in excess of 99% compliance. Joshi *et al.* did not collect data on the percentage of adherence to formularies in their survey.[20] They did ascertain that 10 out of the 60 respondents reported adherence as 'excellent' and a further 22 as 'good'; as mentioned earlier, these were in acute hospitals. The early experience in general practice was of seeking 80–90% adherence to the agreed formulary.[8,9] It can be seen that achieving high adherence is possible, but not without effort. Although the evidence is limited, the impression obtained from looking at formulary development is that, to achieve good adherence, prescribers need to be involved in developing the list, systems are required to keep it updated and feedback to prescribers is necessary. The last point includes both specific intervention by pharmacy staff on an individual basis and general feedback on prescribing patterns.[36] To achieve this, there needs to be an effective pharmacy service with a strong clinical pharmacy presence. If prescriptions do arrive at the dispensary without prior clinical pharmacy review, the dispensary team needs to understand what is required and be prepared to check or challenge the request for non-formulary items.

What of the outcome focused measures, the impact on quality and cost? Chapter 9 addresses the performance management of medicines management, and so explores in more detail what can be meant by 'the quality of prescribing', but here the evidence of the impact of formularies on 'quality', however authors use the term, is considered. The 'impact on cost' is probably a less ambiguous phrase, but it too is imprecise; again the evidence will be examined, whatever the usage.

In looking at the question: 'Do formularies work?', we have already identified some difficulties. The outcomes 'impact on quality' and 'impact on cost' are ill defined. Even the 'intervention itself', the type of formulary system used, can vary enormously in design and in application. Not surprisingly then, the evidence base of the impact of formularies is rather weak. As *Bandolier* put it '[we] expected a large literature and some good literature reviews. We found neither.'[37] They had sought meta-analyses, reviews and randomised controlled trials, using *PubMed* (http://www.ncbi.nlm.nih.gov/entrez/query.fcgi). Following their strategy for the journals they had not covered, no further papers of significance were found. The only randomised controlled trial found was of a single medicine having its range of strengths reduced – hardly very relevant to the complexity of the type of intervention most formulary systems comprise. In an earlier review, the *Drug and Therapeutics Bulletin* concluded that increased quality of prescribing did flow from introducing a formulary, although they noted this was difficult to measure.[13] Avoiding the use of newly introduced medicines that are later withdrawn from the market because of adverse events was seen as a key benefit. This will be returned to later, but presumably there is also a risk of denying access to new medicines that turn out to be significant advances, unless those managing the formulary are consistently prescient.

In the absence of large, randomised controlled trials, what evidence of the impact of formularies is there? George and Hands reported that junior hospital doctors used the information in formularies to shape their prescribing, although how this was measured is not clear from their paper; neither is the extent.[38] If this is correct, a simple list approach to formularies misses an important educational opportunity. Collier and Foster noted their formulary in Wandsworth 'probably improved prescribing by junior staff' and that it reduced risks to patients.[39] The latter assertion was based on the prevention of use of items later withdrawn from the market because of adverse events, evidence used by the

Drug and Therapeutic Bulletin as mentioned earlier. They did not provide any further data that supported the positive safety impact.

Work that provides a little more information on quality is the review by Baker *et al.* of another hospital formulary system.[4] They concluded that their formulary, developed by consensus, did improve the quality of care. Their evidence is limited, concentrating on two therapeutic areas. They reported an overall reduction in non-steroidal anti-inflammatory drug prescribing, particularly marked in accident and emergency care and, presumably, replaced by simple analgesia. No figures were provided on number of prescriptions and no control hospital, not even *post hoc*, was included. Choice of antibiotic was also reported as improved, although the impact was more obvious in terms of finance than quality.

Essex discussed general practice formularies in the *British Medical Journal* in 1989, recommending them as having educational benefits, although accepting that of themselves they do not produce rational prescribing.[40] Once again few data supported the assertions. There are other examples in the literature of the impact of formularies. These include controlling antibiotic use by means of a formulary list or restrictions on specific agents. Usually the 'before and after' approach is taken rather than an independent control. Improved prescribing, fewer adverse events related to therapy and improved antimicrobial sensitivities are reported.[41,42]

It appears, then, that expert opinion and non-controlled studies provide support for the statement that formularies improve the quality of prescribing. One could argue, although formularies could be neutral on improving quality, how could they possibly make prescribing worse? Thus although the experts could be wrong, we have little to lose in terms of prescribing quality – costs could be a separate problem. However, there are ways in which a formulary system could reduce the quality of prescribing. The delayed access to benefits of newly introduced medicines has already been described. Have formulary systems slowed the introduction of atypical antipsychotics or new antiplatelet medicines to the detriment of patients? A second possible problem that a formulary could bring is to lead prescribers into uncritical prescribing – prescribing not in the best interests of individuals and not challenged by pharmacists who are falsely confident because the choice is from the formulary. Thus a doctor may select a formulary product for the 1% of patients who require a non-formulary drug. Alternatively, a formulary medicine may be selected when no treatment would be the best choice. It is appreciated that these examples are not the way formulary systems are intended to work, but without a better evidence base, can we be confident these are not commonplace problems? These hypothetical disbenefits may not be reason to reject the assertion that formularies help to improve the quality of prescribing. However, they should make us critically reflect on our beliefs about the benefits formularies bring.

Having considered the evidence on quality, how do formularies impact on cost? The comment on the lack of major randomised controlled studies applies again. Although there are several examples of formularies having an impact, Collier and Foster reported that their use of a hospital formulary system in the Wandsworth Health Authority reduced the growth in their drug spend.[39] They compared their growth, year on year from 1982 to 1985 to that of the national picture; they found a local increase in spend of 5% per year against a national figure of 12% per year over the same period. Could this be described as reasonable circumstantial evidence with some reservations over the controls? Similarly, a benefit in avoiding growth in spend was reported from general practice in Scotland. A 10–11% saving relative to the rest of Scotland was reported by Beardon et al. when they introduced their formulary in Ninewells.[43] This was achieved through reduced cost per item rather than by prescribing fewer items and related to the period 1981–84.

Work undertaken by Baker et al. in a central London teaching district looked at overall impact and some specific therapeutic areas.[4] During 1980–84, they had a mean annual reduction in overall spend on medicines of 2% after implementing a revised formulary system. The majority of London teaching districts in that period (six out of eight) had an increase of 3% per annum. A large caution is needed here: in the 'intervention' district as well as the formulary there were several other actions to control drug spend. Reductions in outpatient prescribing were made, a programme to reduce waste was implemented and a concerted effort to reduce prices paid for medicines was initiated. It is not clear if any of these were pursued in the other districts. These confounding factors make it difficult to assess the impact of the formulary alone. However, in addition to the gross effect, savings on antibiotics and on non-steroidal anti-inflammatory drugs are reported, which did appear to be linked to the formulary's impact.

Looking more critically at the way formularies are used, Feely et al. compared their hospital's expenditure, during the period after introducing a formulary, to a smaller although similar hospital where an identical formulary was introduced.[36] The key difference in the two sites was the level of feedback; at St James' Hospital (Feely's) feedback on prescribing was given to medical staff, with regular discussions held and detailed information shared. This site saw a fall in cost per patient, whereas the other site saw an 18% rise. Feely *et al.* noted that after the initial gain, costs began to rise again. The key questions – what difference to the subsequent rise and to the cost over the whole period – were not adequately addressed in the report.

A study published in 1996 describing the use of a formulary in general practice in Bedfordshire also provides some evidence of impact on costs.[44] This was a controlled study involving 50 general practitioners in 11 urban and semirural practices in South Bedfordshire, with the remainder of the county (250 general practitioners) as controls. A formulary aimed at covering 80% of cases presented in primary care was developed across the practices involved during the early 1990s. Levels of adherence and impact on cost were assessed; quality was not addressed directly. Data were compared for the first quarter of each calendar year for 1991 (pre-formulary), 1992, 1993 and 1994. Twelve therapeutic groups were included. In just three groups, significant changes in usage patterns occurred: cardiovascular, musculoskeletal and obstetrics and gynaecology. The percentage of generic prescribing rose in the practices where the formulary was introduced and those where it was not: 44% in 1991 in participants, rising to 55% in 1994, 40% in 1990 for controls, rising to 48% in 1994. A similar proportion of practices in both groups became fundholders during the period. The report noted a smaller rise in items prescribed per 'prescribing unit' over the period in the participants than in the controls: 11.8% and 14.0%, respectively. A modest slowing in expenditure growth was also shown, a 41% growth for the formulary practices during 1991–94, a 45% growth for the practices with no formulary over the same period. Using this difference a little cost–benefit modelling was done, with the conclusion that the costs incurred developing the formulary were outweighed by the costs avoided from its application. They estimated break even was achieved after six months, then gains continued throughout the three-year period of the study.

Although there are no large, randomised controlled trials to explore the impact formularies make on the costs and cost-effectiveness of prescribing, the reports described do provide some evidence that costs are controlled, albeit against a background of a steady rise. Certainly if several medicines in a class have similar efficacy and side-effect profiles, but one or two are less costly – perhaps with patents expired – reducing access to the others will, very probably, increase cost-effectiveness. Delaying access to newer agents may also delay the rise in expenditure; thus overall costs in a given period are less than if new agents are immediately used. This does not necessarily increase cost-effectiveness as, of course, benefits of the new drugs are also forgone.

Formulary systems themselves have costs: the decision-making process, the preparation, publishing, implementing, defending perhaps – each uses resources. This, and the lack of confidence regarding their overall impact, mean that there should be an element of doubt in our views regarding the impact of formularies on cost-effectiveness of prescribing. Chapter 7 examines the multifaceted approach to medicines management where the formulary is just one of the elements to control costs and improve quality. It was indeed in that context that the Audit Commission made their assertion, mentioned earlier in this chapter, that the formulary has a key part to play in any medicines management system, supporting cost-effectiveness and quality.

Developing the evidence base

Before concluding this examination of formularies, by considering the 'e-formulary' and proposing the role formularies ought to have, it is worth considering how an evidence base could be, or could have been, developed. Chapter 10 explores the research agenda in more depth.

We have noted that formularies (even when restricting that term's meaning to its usual medicines management context) vary considerably in character, application and coverage. This makes it difficult to undertake a 'controlled experiment' to assess the impact of a defined 'technology'. Perhaps a clinical pharmacology analogy to the question: 'Do formularies work?' is: 'Do cardiovascular medicines work?' – that is, which medicines in what circumstances? Furthermore, as discussed earlier, the question arises: 'What do we mean by work?', once again making 'experiment' design difficult. However, standardised types of formulary and defined outcomes could have been designed and studied. Today, it would be difficult to find a UK healthcare community where there were no current formularies; to set up a first-time introduction of a formulary to explore its impact, while changing from a set list to a guideline-based system, could form the basis of a study.

The reports described in the chapter often had some comparator: the rest of the country or similar hospitals or practices, although these comparators tended not to be well-described. It appeared that confounding was not given much consideration. Historically 'self-controlled' studies, the classic before and after, are well known to be subject to confounding – many other factors change with time, not just the intervention being examined. However, perhaps a combination of these two (similar organisation and before–after) is the best study that is possible without achieving a truly randomised, controlled trial. Indeed, designing a randomised, controlled trial is itself difficult. Randomly allocating patients either to be treated using a formulary or treated with no reference to a formulary, would not be possible. The very process of creating the formulary changes the approach, the understanding and the knowledge of participants; patients in both arms may have their therapy influenced by the intervention being assessed. Random allocation of prescribers or wards to use the formulary would be subject to the same problems. Thus the design would need to be allocation of practices or hospitals or health communities to have the formulary or be the control with no formulary. It is probably too late to undertake such a research project in the UK, although, as mentioned earlier, it might be possible to do so to examine how a major change in a formulary has impact on the various outcomes.

The e-formulary

Information technology can be used to give desktop access to a formulary and to a plethora of guidelines. The prescriber could use the worldwide web or a local network to check whether a specific medicine is available or for the first-line choice in a particular set of circumstances. However, this approach is describing an electronic version of a standard formulary, slightly swifter to access, perhaps. The potential for electronic prescribing systems is much greater. As Slee and Farrar point out: 'Computerised physician entry on-line prescribing can aid formulary management. . . . [It] . . . does facilitate change control and reduces the repetitive parts of formulary management by reminding the prescriber about formulary choices at the time of prescribing'.[45] E-prescribing systems can guide prescribers towards formulary choices by presenting them as the default or easy-access options on menus. In the report from Slee and Farrar, several areas of prescribing were altered by these methods, giving both cost and clinical benefits.

General practice has more commonly had e-prescribing in place than secondary care. A number of systems have been used. PRODIGY (prescribing rationally with decision support in general practice study) is a system developed by the Sowerby Centre for Health Informatics at Newcastle, with support from the Department of Health.[46] The system provides decision support on prescribing. The detailed guidance for medicine choice – the rules followed – was based on an expert panel approach. Some evidence was provided of PRODIGY dampening the growth in spending on medicines, but the validity of these data has been questioned by others.[47–49]

Delaney *et al.*, reviewed the progress on computerised decision support systems in 1999.[50] They concluded that such systems had not delivered the benefits hoped for, although they remained optimistic for the future in this field. Certainly anyone seeking an effective system to manage medicines will need to use the tools that information technology can provide.

The place of the formulary

Having an agreed list of medicines that cover the majority of patient needs on most occasions appears to be a useful part of an organisation's medicines management system. The formulary may be a simple list, perhaps supported by other documents, such as treatment guidelines, but current opinion prefers a more educative document. Although evidence is scarce, intuitively a document that steers prescribing and provides helpful information – particularly in a secondary care setting to support junior doctors – would seem better than a simple list that states what the hospital pharmacy stocks or that general practitioners are expected to have as first choice. It may be that the use of guidelines, discussed in more detail in Chapter 5, means that a physical document called the formulary becomes less relevant. Whether in support of a paper guidelines system or an embedded aspect of an electronic prescribing system, the 'virtual' formulary could become the norm.

Chapter 4 looks at how the entry of new medicines into use can be managed, but formulary 'creation' should be an educative process for those involved and a way of developing commitment to the final document. This would suggest that attempting a formulary for too large a community – multiple primary care trusts and several specialist and hospital trusts – would be problematic. However, it is no longer acceptable for choices on which medicines should be used routinely, to be made by a single organisation in isolation.

Formulary adherence should, in the main, be a self-imposed discipline based on the fact that the majority of situations can properly be dealt with using a medicine from the agreed list. The level of compulsion, or need for senior support for moving off formulary, can be increased in the context of junior doctor prescribing in secondary care. Organisations may wish to include consultant staff in the requirement not to prescribe some items, but a method of dealing with the exceptional patient in exceptional circumstances is necessary. General practitioner freedom to prescribe is enshrined in their conditions of service, but primary care organisations may wish to build incentives or provide feedback to encourage adherence to the agreed selection. However, in both secondary and primary care, effort put in to ensuring that a formulary medicine is chosen should not mean the question: 'Is a prescription needed at all?' is overlooked. No matter how efficient prescribing is, it remains wasteful if no prescription were needed.

A final point, with relation to formularies, is their application in the context of 'patients' own drug schemes'. This is when, on admission to hospital, patients continue to use the medication prescribed and dispensed in primary care. Such schemes have been shown to be cost-saving and are supported within the national medicines management framework.[30,32,51] However, they can involve administration of non-formulary medicines, which could seed other non-formulary prescribing. Having a community-wide formulary helps prevent this potential dilemma. Hospitals need to work with a system that avoids waste, does not expose the patients to avoidable risk and is acceptable to primary care. This may be as simple as using patients' own non-formulary medicines in the short term (many patients will stay less than a week) but being open to a managed switch for longer term patients.

Formularies probably do assist in achieving rational prescribing and help in the pursuit of cost-effective medicine use. They need to have local commitment and relevance, and to be maintained. If this is done, they are a key part of strategic medicines management and can underpin the delivery of pharmaceutical care.

References

1. Critchley M, ed. *Butterworths Medical Dictionary*, 2nd edn, London: Butterworth, 1978.
2. Ministry of Health. *National War Formulary*. London: HMSO, 1941.
3. British Medical Association and the Royal Pharmaceutical Society. *British National Formulary*, 47th edn, London: BMA and RPS, 2004.
4. Baker J, Lant A, Sutters C. Seventeen years' experience of a voluntarily based drug rationalisation programme in hospital. *Br Med J* 1988; 297: 465–469.
5. Middlebrook M. The use of hospital formularies in the UK. *Br J Pharm Pract* 1979; 1: 12–25.
6. Brown A, Barrett C, Herxheimer A. Hospital pharmacy committees in England: their structure, function and development. *Br Med J* 1975; 1: 323–326.
7. Jolles M. Why not compile your own formulary? *Br J Gen Pract* 1981; 31: 372.
8. Green P. The general practice formulary – its role in rational therapeutics. *Br J Gen Pract* 1985; 35: 570–572.

9. Grant G, Gregory D, van Zwanenberg T. Development of a limited formulary for general practice. *Lancet* 1985; 1: 1030–1032.

10. Lothian Liaison Committee. *Lothian Formulary Number 1*. Lothian: LLC, 1987.

11. Royal College of General Practice, Northern Ireland. *Practice Formulary*. Belfast: RCGPNI, 1988.

12. Clucas K (Chair). *Pharmacy: The Report of a Committee of Inquiry Appointed by the Nuffield Foundation*. London: The Nuffield Foundation, 1986.

13. Anon. Local Drug Formularies – are they worth the effort? *Drug and Therapeutics Bulletin* 1989; 27: 13–16.

14. Ridley H. *Drugs of Choice: a Report on the Drug Formularies used in NHS Hospitals*. London: Social Audit, 1986.

15. Petrie J, Scott K. Drug formularies in hospitals. *Br Med J* 1987; 294: 919–920.

16. Department of Health. *The Way Forward for Hospital Pharmaceutical Services* HC 88(54). London: DH, 1988. Also WHC 88(66) (Wales) 1988 and 1988 (GEN) 32 for Scotland 1988.

17. Department of Health. *Health Services Development: Resources, Assumptions and Planning Guidelines* HC (88)43. London: DH, 1988.

18. Harrison P, Standing V, Watling J. *Clinical Pharmacy: a Statement from the Regional Pharmaceutical Officers Committee*. Regional Pharmaceutical Officers, 1988.

19. Greenleaf J, Ellis S, Elliot D, Watling J. *Standards for Pharmaceutical Services in Health Authorities in England*. Regional Pharmaceutical Officers, 1989.

20. Joshi M, Williams A, Petrie J. Hospital formularies in 1993: where and how? *Pharm J* 1994; 253: 63–65.

21. Audit Commission. *A Prescription for Improvement: Towards More Rational Prescribing in General Practice*. London: HMSO, 1994.

22. National Prescribing Centre in conjunction with the NHS Executive. *GP Prescribing Support: a Resource Document and Guide for the New NHS*. NPC and NHSE, 1998.

23. Department of Health. *The New NHS: Modern, Dependable*. London: DH, 1997.

24. Stephens M. Hospital pharmacy within the NHS. In Stephens M, ed. *Hospital Pharmacy* London: Pharmaceutical Press, 2003.

25. Duerden M, Walley T. Prescribing at the interface between primary and secondary care in the UK: towards joint formularies. *Pharmacoeconomics* 1999; 15: 435–443.

26. Richman C. Development of a joint formulary. *Pharm Manage* 2001; 17: 62–63.

27. Crowe S. What you need to do to establish and benefit from a joint formulary. *Med Manage* 2002 1: 20–21.

28. Anon. Interface formulary launched in Birmingham. *Pharm J* 2000; 265: 40.

29. National Prescribing Centre and National Primary Care Research and Development Centre. *Modernising Medicines Management*. Liverpool and Manchester: NPC and NPCRDC, 2002.

30. Department of Health. Medicines management in NHS Trusts: hospital medicines management framework. http://www.dh.gov.uk/PublicationsAnd Statistics/Publications/PublicationsPolicyAndGuidance/PublicationsPolicyAnd

GuidanceArticle/fs/en?CONTENT_ID=4072184&chk=RuVaBK (accessed 15 December 2004).

31. The Scottish Office: NHS in Scotland Management Executive. *Management of the Drugs Bill, NHS Circular MEL (1993)*. Edinburgh: SO, 1993.

32. Audit Commission. *A Spoonful of Sugar: Medicines Management in NHS Hospitals*. London: Audit Commission, 2001.

33. Southampton and South West Hampshire Health Authority, Working Party on Antibiotics. *Antibiotic Guidelines for use in Adults Only*. Southampton: SSWHHA, 1978.

34. Southampton and South West Hampshire Health Authority, Drug and Therapeutics Sub-committee. *Limited Drugs List for Hospital Use*. Southampton: SSWHHA, 1985.

35. Wessex Regional Health Authority. *Wessex Formulist*. Winchester: Wessex RHA, 1993.

36. Feely J, Chan R, Cocoman L *et al.* Hospital formularies: need for continuous intervention. *Br Med J* 1990; 300: 28–30.

37. Do formularies work? *Bandolier* [Apr 2002; 98-5]. http://www.jr2.ox.ac.uk/bandolier/band98/b98-5.html (accessed 8 December 2004).

38. George C, Hands D. Drug and therapeutic committees and information pharmacy services: the United Kingdom. *World Dev* 1983; 11: 229–236.

39. Collier J, Foster J. Management of a rational drugs policy in hospital. The first five years' experience. *Lancet* 1985; 1: 331–333.

40. Essex B. Practice formularies: towards rational prescribing. *Br Med J* 1989; 298: 1052.

41. Climo M, Israel D, Wong E *et al.* Hospital-wide restriction of clindamycin: effect on the incidence of *Clostridium difficile* associated diarrhoea and cost. *Ann Intern Med* 1998; 128: 989–995.

42. Vlahovic-Palcevski V, Morovic M, Palceuski G. Antibiotic utilization at the university hospital after introducing an antibiotic policy. *Eur J Clin Pharmacol* 2000; 56: 97–101.

43. Beardon P, Brown S, Mowat D *et al.* Introducing a drug formulary to a general practice; effects on prescribing costs. *Br J Gen Pract* 1987; 37: 305–307.

44. Hill-Smith I. Sharing resources to create a district drug formulary: a county-wide controlled trial. *Br J Gen Pract* 1996; 46: 271.

45. Slee A, Farrar K. Formulary management – effective computer management systems. *Pharm J* 1999; 262: 363–365.

46. Department of Health. What is PRODIGY? http://www.prodigy.nhs.uk/AboutProdigy/WhatisProdigy.asp (accessed 15 December 2004).

47. NHS Executive. PRODIGY *Phase One*. London: NHSE, 1998.

48. NHS Executive. PRODIGY *Phase Two*. London: NHSE, 1998.

49. Buchan I, Hanka R, Penchean D, Bundred P. Introduction of the computer assisted prescribing scheme Prodigy was premature. *Br Med J* 1996; 313: 1083.

50. Delaney B, Fitzmaurice D, Riaz A, Hobbs F. Can computerised decision support systems deliver improved quality in primary care? *Br Med J* 1999; 319: 1281–1283.

51. Dua S. Establishment and audit of a patients' own drug scheme. *Hosp Pharm* 2000; 7: 196–198.

4

Managed entry of medicines

Decision making is an activity embedded in medicines management, both at the level of the individual patient and at a strategic level. Of course, 'to prescribe or not to prescribe' should be a question for regular consideration, perhaps every time a prescription is written, but this chapter explores some of the processes around decision making for strategic medicines management.

Chapter 3 looks at the formulary and the fact that there is limited evidence of their impact. Chapter 6 explores how guidelines are developed and used. In both activities an examination of evidence is essential; this chapter addresses how the evidence can be used, not only for new medicines but also for established therapeutic groups. It is clear that managing new medicines, and use of older ones, are informed by national guidance; this is explored in Chapter 1. However, considerable work remains necessary at organisational or local community level. The important financial planning processes tied into managed entry are discussed in Chapter 8.

Why manage entry?

There are various controls on the production, marketing and use of medicines. The Medicines Act and the Misuse of Drugs Act are two obvious examples. The majority of prescriptions are for medicines that are 'licensed' for use, with marketing authorisation given by the Medicines and Healthcare Products Regulatory Agency (MHRA).[1] The MHRA sees that medicines, which meet the standards of safety, quality and efficacy, are provided with this marketing authorisation before they can be prescribed or sold, although 'unlicensed' products are prescribable. The MHRA carries out pre-marketing assessment of the medicine's safety, quality and efficacy, by reviewing trial and other data, before a decision is made on whether the product should be granted a marketing authorisation. So, with this in place, why should organisations be concerned about controlling the entry of medicines and, indeed, the managed access to medicines throughout their life cycle? Not surprisingly, in line with this book's theme, the answer suggested here is twofold: risk to patients and risk to financial control.

Large numbers of new preparations arrive on the market each year, with significant numbers of additional drugs – perhaps many of the 'me too' variety. Edition 46 of the *British National Formulary* included 27 new preparations; edition 47 has 26 additions.[2,3] Along with demographic change and increasing expectations, the availability of new technologies, in this case, medicines, is a significant pressure on health service financing. There is also an argument that these new medicines are small steps at big costs. To put it in economic terms – we are experiencing diminishing marginal utility. The 20th century discovery of penicillin, chlorpromazine and of the use of insulin gave big benefits for small costs, whereas the arrival of more sophisticated agents in recent years gives limited benefits at big costs. This is a gross oversimplification of matters but is relevant when, for example, a fourth or fifth medicine is considered in a risk-reducing regimen for cardiovascular therapy. We ought to note that some of the increased costs of medicines are due to the more stringent regulation – there are costs incurred if we wish to avoid bringing a highly teratogenic drug to market.

In 2002 Garattini and Bertele pointed out that, of cancer medicines, 'the costs of new preparations are several times higher than existing drugs', when they are 'largely equivalent to the standard treatments in efficacy and safety.'[4] Examples they used included moving to topotecan from cisplatin and use of liposomal doxorubicin. The latter, they argued, was marketed as being safer owing to reduced cardiotoxicity, when in fact cardiotoxicity was never a particular problem in clinical practice.

The issue of marketing and, more narrowly, advertising is of great relevance to managing medicines. Evidence-based medicine could be seen as way to improve practice from that based on personal experience and anecdote, but perhaps the true value of evidence-based medicine is to act as a counterbalance to 'advert-led-prescribing'. Work in the United States found that, in 1998, nearly $13,000 million dollars were spent by the pharmaceutical industry on promoting products within the country, with nearly 52% spent on just 50 drugs.[5] Of course, these figures include significant expenditure on direct-to-consumer promotion. By 2003 the total spend was quoted as $19,000 million dollars.[6] Although it would hardly be reasonable simply to say 'they wouldn't do it if it didn't work', especially in a chapter promoting an evidence-based approach, it is strongly tempting to say just that. Wolfe certainly argued that pharmaceutical industry promotion is in part responsible for poor prescribing.[7] Kessler suggested that needless injury or even death has resulted from physicians being persuaded to use products 'in ways not adequately tested' – safety is a theme to be revisited later.[8]

Having dwelt on the 'downside', it is fair to state a contrary case. Without new medicines there would be no new benefits – irrespective of the marginal utility. Calfee, from the American Enterprise Institute, argues that pharmaceutical marketing has benefits.[9] The prize of profit from a new medicine is increased by the ability to market it; hence the incentive to develop is greater and so marketing helps drive up opportunities for health gain. He also points out that promotion gets information to prescribers, reducing the time lag of evidence to practice. There is some logic in this, but marketing, promotion and advertising allowed free rein, with no counterbalancing evidence appraisal, controlled entry and, indeed, strategic medicines management, could result in organisations having no ability to control finances.

So far the focus has been on finance and, in particular, the pressure caused by marketing. Before moving to risk, it is worth noting that without marketing, there would still be pressure to use new agents or expand the use of old agents. If a magic curtain could be put up around a health community allowing in only critically appraised evidence of high quality and preventing all but the beneficial influence of pharmaceutical companies, there would still be an enthusiasm for the new. Why? One could create a long list of reasons – curiosity, scientific enquiry, desperation, but the most obvious is that healthcarers genuinely wish to see patients derive benefit from treatments, preferably with fewer side-effects than the current medicines produce. However, resources are finite and there are competing demands, so managing entry and controlled access would still be required.

Turning from finances to patient safety, is this a valid second reason to pursue managing medicines? Kessler, mentioned earlier, implied this is so.[8] Chapter 3 gives examples from the literature where a formulary reduced access to a new medicine and, the authors believed, prevented untoward events. Benoxaprofen was one such medicine. Although there are differing views on how benoxaprofen's arrival resulted in so many adverse events, Geoffrey Tucker's comments at the 1995 Pharmaceutical Conference gives a very pertinent view for this chapter.[10] He argued that key in the 'Opren tragedy' was a pharmacokinetic problem: benoxaprofen achieves much higher plasma concentrations in the frail elderly than in younger patients – especially healthy volunteers used for the initial work. By implication then, had benoxaprofen been used more cautiously and the frail elderly not exposed, it might have had a longer, less problematic shelf-life.

Temple and Himmel's editorial in the *Journal of the American Medical Association* in May 2002, discusses the issues of new medicines and the fact that premarketing trials can never reveal all the possible adverse events.[11] They comment on the paper by Lasser *et al.* that examined medicines coming to market between 1975 and 1999.[12] Lasser *et al.* predicted that 20% of new chemical entities brought to market would later be withdrawn or have additional warnings added. This figure is thought by Temple and Himmel to overstate the case – early 'disclosure' of adverse events having improved by the late 1990s. However, they still conclude that prescribers need to think very carefully when starting a recently introduced medicine. This is reinforced by recent events around the use of antidepressants, for example the MHRA warning on venlafaxine use for children and adolescents.[13] Extending use to this group, beyond the market authorisation, was found to have no great benefit but carried additional risks, including that of increased suicidal ideation and hostility. Although not wishing to imply that prescribers recklessly introduce new medicines, these events and arguments do suggest that, irrespective of finances, new medicines should receive the attention of organisations and that managed entry has an important safety role.

There are two further aspects relating to safety, one to the products themselves and one to prescribing responsibility. *Building a Safer NHS for Patients: Improving Medication Safety* states that 'assessment of potential risks associated with the labelling and packaging of products should be a routine part of NHS procurement processes.'[14] Choosing medicines, controlling entry and access, should take into account the products and the medication, not just the medicine. It may seem absurd to prohibit use of a particular medicine just because the packaging or name is similar to another, but if there really is a problem and substituting another medicine would solve it, then why not? Safety of the medication should form part of the consideration when controlling entry; this could mean a new agent is readily supported because it solves a safety problem.

Prescribing responsibility was also mentioned. Managing entry and controlling access can use prescriber restrictions as tools to control use, that is, some doctors are allowed prescribe but others are asked not to. However, from another perspective, active management of medicine entry could be seen as the responsible way of preventing confusion over who should take on prescribing of a new medicine – a reason for managed entry. Shared care arrangements are explored further in the Chapter 7.

In summary then, managing the entry and use of medicines is a response to the need to control finances and is part of our responsibility to protect patients. Before looking at the various steps in the process and the evidence of their impact, it is worth examining the life cycle of medicines and considering the different responses that are required for the various stages.

A medicine's life cycle

There are various ways to describe the history of a particular medicine. The perspective of a shareholder could be taken, perhaps beginning with a period of hope that pushes up the pharmaceutical company's share price, followed by fulfilment and sustained value or by disillusion accompanying significant fall. Here the perspective of an organisation seeking to manage medicines will be taken: chemical entities are discovered, developed, some are brought to trial as medicines, marketed, then may be copied, improved upon or seen just not to deliver the expected benefits. Other than the very early stages, strategic medicines management requires some action by organisations at each step.

New drugs may be derived from a natural source – plant or animal or mineral – may be synthesised chemically or created using biotechnology. The motivation to produce compounds that can be developed into medicines could be described as a desire to solve a problem. The problem could be a disease with no adequate treatment, a 'new' disease or a disease where current therapy is failing, such as increased resistance to anti-infectives. Similarly, the problem could be that a medicine is effective but prone to side-effects, so a cleaner product is required. Another view on motivation is that compounds are sought to produce medicines that will sell, with adaptations made to products just before the patent on the 'parent' product expires. Certainly the *NHS Plan* is positive about the role of pharmaceutical and bio-pharmaceutical industry – 'a UK success story' – and makes clear that they are vital in the development of new medicines that can bring benefits to patients.[15] The DH-produced plan also made clear the desire that research was speedy, with efficient ethics committees and enhanced recruitment to trials.

Harman describes the development process in overview in a helpful summary in the *Pharmaceutical Journal*.[16] Figure 4.1 presents his figures on the ratio of new compounds to those coming to market (10,000 to 1)

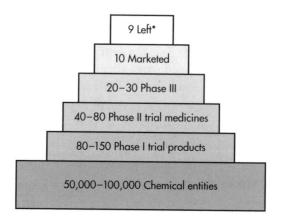

Figure 4.1 From compounds to medicines: diminishing numbers. Note that of the nine compounds left, a very small percentage of medicines are withdrawn but 10% may have significant changes to marketing authorisation (based on Lasser et al.[12]).

and builds in the figures from Lasser's work, mentioned earlier. The initial work on screening the compounds will be *in vitro*; pharmacological but also chemical and physical properties are investigated. As the number of compounds reduces, so the journey towards clinical testing begins. More *in vitro* models, such as tests on human cells, are being sought to minimise the need for animal studies, but considerable preclinical work in animals is required. Toxicology, carcinogenicity and teratogenicity are explored before humans are exposed to the new product. Work on the pharmaceutical aspects – how the medicine will be developed and presented – is also undertaken.

Phase I clinical studies are the first step involving human exposure. Typically between 50 and 100 healthy volunteers are exposed to the putative medicine. The aim is to test effect and increase the dose towards the expected clinical use to observe any adverse effect. Efficacy is not being explored since there is no disease. Phase II clinical studies then follow. These involve patients with the disease or condition being treated. Various dosing regimens are tried. For most compounds numbers treated will be greater than 100 but fewer than 500, although for rare conditions such numbers may not be feasible. Efficacy is being explored at this stage.

The next stage in a medicine's life cycle is the phase III clinical trial. Here, several thousand patients will be included. Ideally, randomised entry, double blinded, comparative trials will be undertaken, using the 'gold standard' therapy as comparator. Some crossover element may be appropriately added to improve the design. Clearly, where the treatment offered is novel there may be no active comparator so a placebo is appropriate. The size of a trial required to demonstrate the benefit of the medicine will depend on the size of the effect sought and the natural variability of the measures made. During the phase III trial period, there may be some non-trial compassionate use. This will tend to be limited to specialists in centres of expertise and will be organised on a named patient basis. At the later stages of phase III work, an application for authorisation to market will be made, for the very few compounds left under consideration. The more cynical may argue that the marketing has already begun, with participation of clinicians in trials and the issue of information, albeit in a very controlled way, to budget holders and so on.

The next stage is regulatory approval and market launch. Considerable effort is put in by the pharmaceutical industry to get information to key influencers at time of launch and to get a slice of market share. After marketing, the wider use of the medicine will inevitably lead to reports of further adverse events, as mentioned above. The Committee on Safety of Medicines' yellow card scheme is used to report all adverse events on newly launched medicines, as well as all serious events throughout a medicine's life cycle. Phase IV postmarketing trial work will also continue.

For most novel medicines, there soon follow a number of other compounds marketed with claims of better efficacy, or fewer side-effects, or no interactions, or easier to swallow, or some other unique selling point. This is a new stage for a medicine and to which organisations must respond. Comparative effectiveness becomes a key issue; pragmatic clinical trials and economic analyses may become particularly useful.

Assuming the medicine has survived each stage described so far, there remain two possible further stages: continued usefulness with loss of patent or genuine redundancy owing to development of a replacement (or disappearance of the disease perhaps). A medicine might move through each or remain a useful generic medicine for the long term. Paracetamol is, perhaps, a prime example of the latter. At or around the start of these stages an innovative pharmaceutical company may well develop an adapted version of their medicine – modified release perhaps. This could be seen as squeezing extra benefits for patients from their entrepreneurial endeavours or as trying to keep the profits going as long as possible. If seen as the latter, then who could dispute the reasoning, as Harman estimates, that by the 1990s as much as £350 million is spent in getting from basic science to market launch of a single medicine.

Before moving on from the life cycle to examine some of the

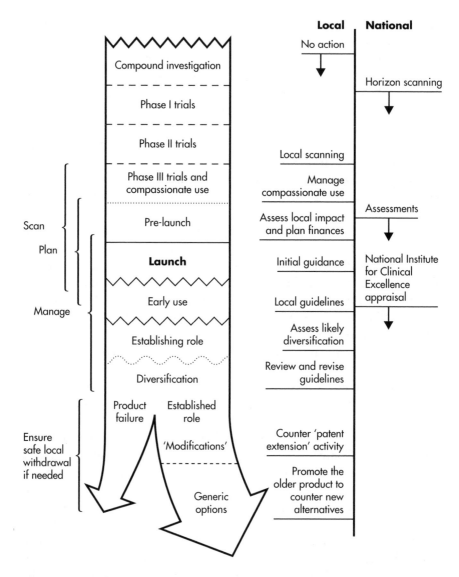

Figure 4.2 Medicines management activities along the medicine's life cycle.

strategic medicines management activities in detail, it is worth summarising how these need to keep pace with the development process. Figure 4.2 attempts to map the medicines management activity against the life cycle stages. The basic science and early discovery work probably merit little attention from local organisations, although national or academic bodies may wish to note what patents have been sought. Phase

II and III monitoring will begin to feed into organisation plans, particular in centres committed to significant trial work. Appraisal, local impact assessment and planning will need to be in place as marketing authorisation is sought. A clear plan of action needs to be in place at time of marketing, although this may be to do nothing if the medicine is considered to be of little risk financially or clinically. Decisions by relevant committees, dissemination of guidance and financial planning should be ready if the organisation wants to manage entry rather than hope that advert-led prescribing either doesn't happen or, if it does, that it is beneficial and affordable.

The later stages of the medicine's life cycle may require a different kind of intervention. Once a medicine becomes generic, the big promotion stops. This could allow the primary care trust pharmacist to relax and count the savings, such as with fluoxetine, but actually may require some measures to counter the drift to more heavily promoted medicines that remain on patent at premium price. Finally an action might be to warn prescribers actively against use of a medicine found to be of little benefit or where a newer therapy is safer. Withdrawals of medicines usually occur with considerable publicity, so the role there may be simply to ensure that sound advice as to what to move on to is available.

Scanning, planning and managing

Brzezicki describes horizon scanning as 'the new mantra' and points to the NPC's support for PCT pharmacists in this activity.[17] However, he does note the difficulties posed by the uncertainty of the impact of even well-scanned developments, since foreknowledge of price is rare. Horizon scanning is not a new activity but it is a key feature of strategic medicines management, whatever its limitations. Crucially, scanning needs to be linked to planning and managing; it is not an end in itself for PCT-led pharmacists or trust chief pharmacists. Simply to know that in the coming year a high-cost therapy for a relatively common haematological cancer is likely to be marketed and to do nothing about it, is no better than to be surprised by its launch. Horizon scanning can enable planning and prepare local health communities for managing medicines as they arrive and move into use.

Medicines information services have had an important role in horizon scanning for many years.[18] This has evolved as collaboration with the NPC has developed and with the arrival of NICE. Collaboration between medicines information services and the National Horizon Scanning Centre (NHSC) is also well-established.

The NHSC is based in the Health Management Centre at Birmingham University; it is described as 'a joint collaboration between the Department of Health and Epidemiology and the Health Economics Facility' of the university.[19] The NHSC identifies medicines in development and begins to describe their likely impact. Their website details briefings on new and emerging technologies. An example of a briefing from 2003 is a therapy in development for ovarian cancer: $_{90}$Y-muHMFG1.[20] This work probably is of only passing direct interest to local organisations but it is a vital feeder for further national work. The NHSC works with the UK Medicines Information Group (UKMi) to produce details of medicines in development for prioritisation for review, supporting the NPC Prioritisation Group.

Since 2003 the NPC, UKMi and its network of medicines information centres have produced a revised set of documents to support the scanning/planning/managing process for medicines. Table 4.1 summarises these. Details are available via the NPC and UKMi websites, but NHS net connection is required for specific documents.[21] *Prescribing Outlook – August 2003 Part A*, a document confidential to the NHS, provided information on medicines expected to be launched over the subsequent 12–18 months.[22] New medicines and medicines expected to have revised indications are included. *Prescribing Outlook – October 2003 Part B*, is a UKMi-produced document, led by the London–South Thames Medicines Information Centre, again confidential to the NHS, that estimates the impact of national policy and guidance plus the expected impact of important trials that are due to report.[23] These two documents (updated editions of which were published in 2004) can form the basis of work undertaken at a local level in identifying the expected pressures for the coming year. Chapter 8 discusses the financial planning cycle where this work must be applied.

More detail on specific developments is given in the other NPC/UKMi documents. *New Drugs in Clinical Development* monographs are concise reviews of new medicines that are expected to receive NICE appraisals at launch. They are issued about a year prior to launch. *On the Horizon, Future Medicines* arrive about six months before a product launch and are aimed at medicines unlikely to receive a NICE review or, if to be reviewed, the review will not be available immediately after marketing begins. The Wessex Drug and Medicines Information Centre and the Newcastle Drug and Therapeutics Centre work with the NPC on these documents. *On the Horizon, Rapid Review* is planned as an update to these initial bulletins and is prepared in the first three months after marketing. The UKMi website (www.ukmi.nhs.uk) has a specific, controlled-access section called *New Drugs Online* that

Table 4.1 National Prescribing Centre UK Medicines Information Group documents

Title	Notes	When produced
New Drugs in Clinical Development (monographs)	Each one is a review of a medicine coming to market which NICE is expected to appraise at an early stage	Around 12 months before launch
On the Horizon (Future Medicines Bulletin)	Each is a review of a medicine coming to market which NICE will not appraise or not appraise at an early stage	Around 6 months before launch
On the Horizon (rapid review)	Updates the Future Medicines Bulletin where this is required	In the first 3 months after marketing
On the Horizon (newsletter)	Regular update on new medicines	As required, several times each year
New Medicines on the Market	Concise evaluations of newly marketed medicines	In the first 3 months after launch
Therapeutic Overview	Broad overview that summarises developments in a particular therapeutic area	As required
Prescribing Outlook (Part A and Part B)	Summary of expected developments (A) and of the expected impact of national guidance (B)	Annually between August and October

NICE = National Institute of Clinical Excellence.

provides information on medicines from phase II trials to post-launch; it also has links to the various items already described here.

These various documents, supplemented by local tailoring, assist the financial planning process as already mentioned. In addition there is an opportunity to begin to plan the local agenda for prescribing and therapeutic committees. The developments with biggest impact will need space at committee meetings and, unless national documents cover the necessary ground and arrive in timely fashion, also time for local appraisal to inform the decision-making process. Chapter 2 describes the typical committee structures, which do vary in detail, but have the fundamental role in guiding the use of medicines.

Informed by horizon-scanning documents and with financial and agenda planning in place, the final aspect is the managing of medicines. Before the launch of a product, some decision making may be necessary: what to do about patients experiencing new medicines but in a trial setting which ends before launch, how to handle compassionate use outside the trial context. The former should be dealt with by the trial protocol. The latter is more difficult. A simple refusal may mean benefits for individuals are missed; an open approach could expose patients to risks and organisations to the uncontrolled introduction of medicines.

Around launch, local committees may wish to restrict access to the medicine by advising that only certain groups of prescribers may use them. In some cases they may wish to encourage no use at all, until an appropriate assessment is undertaken and, if use is approved, the financial support put in place. Chapter 3 considers the role of formularies in restricting access; the remainder of this chapter looks at how evidence can be used and how decisions can be made.

Do we want this new medicine?

Although the basic approach will be similar, there will be differences in how various groups of new medicines are tackled. The differences are in terms of comparators, importance and ability to restrict. A medicine may be novel – the first of a class to treat a disease or symptom where nothing effective was previously available, although this is increasingly rare. A new medicine may be novel but in a therapeutic area where medicines from other classes are already in use. The medicine may be an agent of the 'me too' kind, a new chemical entity but second, third, fourth or later of the class already in use – another angiotensin-converting enzyme inhibitor or proton pump inhibitor. Finally, the medicine may be a modified version of a product already in use – a sustained release version, combination product or even an isomer. The earlier items in the list may prove harder to rank in importance as comparators are just not available; refusal may also be difficult even if seen as desirable. The later groups probably have greater data and, whether chosen to replace older products or their use restricted, limiting access may be considerably easier.

Whichever group is under consideration, the hurdles medicines can be required to jump for access to be supported follow the same pattern:

- Does the medicine work? (Efficacy)
- What are the outcomes in 'real life'? (Effectiveness)
- How do the outcomes compare with the costs? (Cost-effectiveness)
- Have we the funds to obtain the potential benefits? (Affordability)

The four steps – efficacy, effectiveness, cost-effectiveness and affordability – are usually dealt with as different stages. Efficacy can be assumed by market authorisation – phase II and phase III studies show the medicine has an effect. Effectiveness has been defined as 'the extent to which an intervention produces a beneficial outcome in the routine

Table 4.2 Features of explanatory and pragmatic trials

Feature	Explanatory trial	Pragmatic trial
What is explored?	Efficacy	Effectiveness
Exclusion criteria	Extensive and strict	Permissive
Population included	Carefully selected to address issue of effect	Natural, 'real life' to test what will happen in practice
Subjects included in analysis of results	Only those actually receiving the intervention	All, on an 'intention to treat' basis
Focus of study	The intervention	The context as well as the intervention
Controls used	Placebo or alternative therapy	Standard therapy
Problems	May not be generalisable	May have confounding factors

setting.'[24] Phase III, randomised controlled trials can provide insight into effectiveness, but the more telling evidence will come from pragmatic studies rather than those that are explanatory, that is, those with idealised circumstances. Table 4.2 summarises the key features of explanatory and pragmatic studies – the extremes are stated, many trials fall in the middle ground. The data to answer the outcomes versus costs question will come from health economic modelling at first, then from economic analyses built into or alongside pragmatic trials. Chapter 5 explores health economic issues. Affordability questions can only be dealt with by local organisations and health communities and will always involve making choices. At the risk of using some cumbersome clichés – the bottom line is, that no matter how efficacious or effective or how big a bang you get for your buck, with no buck to spare you won't hear anything.

A well-known schematic for placing a new therapy is shown in Figure 4.3. It lays out a grid comparing a new medicine with one already on the market. Items falling into the upper right hand box are, by definition, more cost-effective than the comparator – they are cheaper and more effective. Such medicines are not too common, but are easy choices if they are marketed. Items in the lower left hand box are more costly and less effective – if they ever do get launched, they are not too difficult to reject. Medicines in the other boxes (and those on the lines) are where difficult decisions need to be made and where most new therapies can be placed.

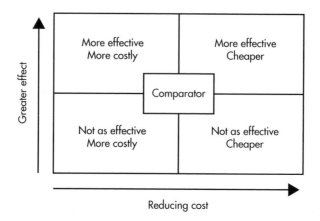

Figure 4.3 Schematic to place a new medicine.

Figure 4.4 adds a further dimension: safety, or the side-effect profile. This is more difficult to visualise but the comparator is in the centre with the 'best' box being the safer, cheaper, better cube at the top, deep right. Again new medicines fall into the decision boxes – perhaps more effective, but with a greater cost and a worse side-effect profile and so on. Whichever model is preferred, managing entry of new medicines will involve two phases: looking at the evidence to find out where the medicine fits in comparison with available treatments; and making a decision about trading off the features because it is unlikely that it will sit at the extremes.

Evidence-based decisions

Having set out the crude parameters, the next section will examine how evidence-based decisions can be made in the context of medicines management. Evidence-based medicine has been defined by Sackett *et al.* as 'the conscientious, explicit and judicious use of current best evidence in making decisions about the care of individual patients.'[25] For strategic medicines management, an evidence-based approach is the use of the appropriate, up-to-date evidence to inform decisions around access to and use of medicines for a local health community or organisation. An evidence-based approach can also apply to the processes and systems used, although as can been seen in other chapters, evidence for medicines management systems is often sparse. There has been a considerable literature on the evidence-based approach in recent years,

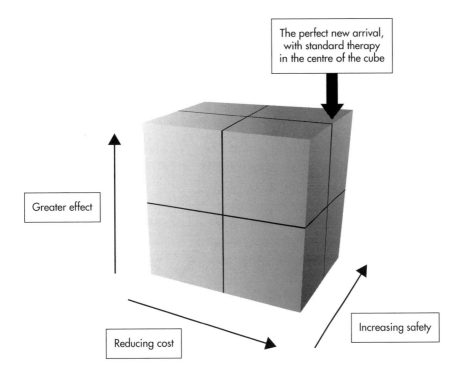

Figure 4.4 Schematic to place a new medicine, including safety.

in the medical and pharmaceutical press and in texts.[24,26–30] Here I will concentrate on the types of evidence, appraising the evidence, presenting the evidence and coming to a decision.

Types of evidence

Moore and McQuay, in 1997, described a five-tier hierarchy of evidence, from the most reliable to the least, based on the design or nature of the source.[31] NICE has a six-tier hierarchy and, although omitting expert opinion, Jones reports a seven-tier pyramid of evidence.[29,30] For convenience, the NICE hierarchy will be used here. Table 4.3 summaries this. Chapter 6 revisits evidence-grading in the context of guideline production.

Systematic reviews

Whichever classification system is chosen, the gold standard for evidence will be a good, systematic review of well-designed, controlled,

Table 4.3 The evidence hierarchy[31]

Level	Description
1a	Systematic review of evidence, including meta-analysis, derived from randomised controlled trials of good design, with appropriate power
1b	Evidence from one or more well-designed, randomised controlled trials
2a	Evidence from controlled trials of good design but not with randomised entry
2b	Evidence from quasi-experimental study or studies
3	Evidence from well-designed, non-experimental studies: cohort studies, case control studies
4	Evidence based on expert opinion or case reports

1a = Most reliable; 4 = least reliable.

randomised entry trials. Khan *et al.* define a systematic review as a research article that identifies relevant studies, appraises their quality and summarises their results using a scientific methodology.[24] Their text gives a good explanation of such reviews and the summarising techniques that can be employed, although it would be easy, if examining their definition only, to interpret the term 'scientific methodology' quite narrowly as meaning meta-analysis or other statistical technique. In fact, systematic review outputs may not always lend themselves to such techniques. Systematic reviews can be undertaken with or without meta-analysis – the terms are not synonymous. However, meta-analysis, where appropriate, is a helpful way to combine trial data to produce a straightforward summary of effect.

The starting point for a systematic review is identifying the question to be pursued. Systematic reviews should state their purpose, then choose a methodology to achieve it. Khan *et al.* describe a systematised approach to question generation, moving from a vague enquiry to a question specifying the population to be included, the intervention to be examined and the outcome being sought from the intervention.[24]

A formally planned literature search, which enables the researcher to find all the relevant literature, should then be followed. This is where systematic is important; editorial reviews or texts that draw on the literature without covering it all, may be informative but are prone to bias. Authors of such non-systematic reviews may veer towards papers that support their inclinations; for community-prescribing decisions and for guidelines, this is not likely to be acceptable. Incomplete searches, irrespective of the authors' prejudices, may also result in misleading conclusions; important data may be missed or the weight of the evidence understated. There will need to be not only a process of weeding out irrelevant or unsuitable papers but also to check for completeness in terms of hard-to-find sources and papers that arrive in press during the review process.

Systematic reviews should assess the quality of the evidence found and, when presented, state how this has been done. Wiffen gives an example of a scoring system where a score of 0 to 5 can be achieved based on trial design and how withdrawals are addressed.[28] Khan *et al.* advise that a minimum quality threshold should be set at the selection stage of the literature search, then a detailed checklist relevant to the question should be made to test the studies that remain under consideration.[24] In this section of the book, systematic reviews of randomised controlled trials are being examined as the best source of evidence; thus the relevant minimum standard would be that such a design was used. For other purposes, systematic reviews may be carried including studies of less rigorous design.

Having found and assessed the literature, the systematic reviewer's next step is to summarise the evidence. This will involve collation and tabulation of findings plus the careful summation or synthesis of evidence where this is possible. Within this process there is a danger of summating effects of an intervention to provide a conclusion when in fact the individual studies do not warrant summation – heterogeneity exists. An example of this would be where a medicine is used in three studies, each well-designed but having very different populations; the individual results may show a large positive effect in two trials but no effect in the third; crude summation would suggest a moderate effect for everyone. Thus a result is obtained which misleads for all three populations. With this word of caution, summation and synthesis should be viewed as key to gaining insight into the question posed by the reviewer.

Meta-analysis is a statistical technique that combines results from individual trials to give an overall result. Weighting is given to each study so that the result is influenced more by the 'better' studies. Khan *et al.* suggest the weighting is usually based on the inverse of the variance in each study – the greater the variance the less weight is place on the trial.[24] There are, however, two distinct approaches to combining results – a fixed-effect model and a random-effects model. The former assumes the individual trials each give an answer that approximates to the correct answer; it weights larger studies preferentially. The latter, random-effects model, assumes there is a distribution of correct answers – because studies are not all equivalent – and it weights smaller studies favourably. This means small studies 'punch above their weight', having a relatively greater impact on the result, rather than an absolutely greater impact than does a large study. Software packages are available to assist the combination and display of results.

The literature has many examples of meta-analysis used to summarise results of systematic review. The Antithrombotic Trialists' Collaboration reported their meta-analysis of antiplatelet therapy effects in the *British Medical Journal* in 2002; it provides a good example of this type of research.[32] Their work combined 287 studies, exploring the impact of antiplatelet therapy on occlusive vascular events in patients at high risk of such problems. Results provided included the absolute reductions in risk, comparative reductions from different agents and comparison of extra protection with risk of adverse events. Another *British Medical Journal* meta-analysis from 2002 is the Furukawa *et al.* report of the effects and side-effects of low-dose tricyclic antidepressants.[33] They report their use of the random effects model on the grounds of ease of interpretation and generalisability; they used 'review manager' software to assist analysis. The methods allowed the authors to make conclusions that, they state, added to knowledge. In this case the fact that, although lower-dose tricyclics may or may not be as efficacious as higher doses, the drop-out rate caused by side-effects is much lower and hence low-dose tricyclics merit consideration as a therapeutic tool.

The two examples given here both use pictorial representations of the results, in what Davies and Crombie call 'blobbograms'.[34] The blobbogram, or Forest plot, shows each trial and the summary result on a chart. Figure 4.5 is an example of such a plot. The size of a dot or square can indicate size of trial (or weighting), and confidence interval (typically 95%) is shown by a horizontal line. The aggregate effect is also indicated. The plot is of odds ratio or of relative risk, for which a logarithmic scale is used.

Meta-analysis is a tool that helps to summarise results. Whether this tool or other means are chosen, the final stages of a systematic review are to interpret the findings and present conclusions. Khan *et al.* suggest that reviewers check their results for selection bias at this stage, with the funnel plot being one possible technique.[24] In essence a funnel plot is a diagram showing each of the individual trial results, one axis for size of trial, the other for size of effect. Figure 4.6 gives an example. The name 'funnel' derives from the expected shape: a good review will have a plot with a wide bottom and a narrow top, demonstrating that small trials give a wide spread around the true result, and large trials a narrow spread around the true result. Where literature has been missed

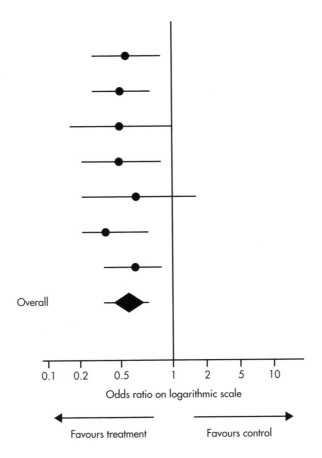

Figure 4.5 Plotting results of meta-analysis.

or not published, the funnel will have gaps. The gaps are most likely to fall at the little or no effect end of the plot; this is described as publication bias and is thought to be due to the reluctance of sponsors, authors and editors to publish trials that show interventions to have failed. However, Wiffen notes that this notion of symmetry in plot, meaning no bias, is subject to challenge.[28] Davies and Crombie suggest another method in addition; they propose calculating the number of negative trials of a given size (ones contrary to the summarised result) that would be needed to 'neutralise' the effect demonstrated, the idea being that if a ridiculously large number would be required, then the reviewers would not feasibly have missed them all.[34]

After a selection-bias check, reviewers should comment on the overall strength and weaknesses of the evidence, state whether the

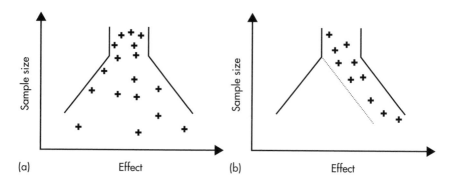

Figure 4.6 The funnel plot. Each plus sign is a trial result. (a) Symmetry implying unbiased publication. (b) Asymmetry implying possible publication bias.

results apply to some or to all the potential populations and give a meaningful summary of the effect found. The final point would normally be the statement of an odds ratio or statement of relative risk, as mentioned above. The odds ratio is the figure derived from dividing the chance of an outcome in the experimental group by the chance of that outcome in the control group. Thus an odds ratio of 1 means the intervention is no different from the control, a ratio above 1 means the intervention is more likely to give the outcome than the control, whereas if below 1 then the intervention is less likely to cause the outcome than the control. Relative risk is the ratio of risk in the experimental group to that in the control group. Wiffen gives a useful summary of the differences between odds ratios and relative risks in *Evidence-based Pharmacy*, the key points being that although odds ratios are mathematically superior, they are harder to interpret.[28] A third way to summarise and report findings is to state the number needed to treat; this is straightforward and accessible. Its use is explored later in the chapter in the context of decision making. It states the number of patients who would need to be treated, over a specified time period, for the desired outcome to be achieved; it is derived from the reciprocal of the absolute risk reduction.

Systematic reviews undertaken to high standards are the top level of the evidence hierarchy, but they are still subject to problems. Wiffen suggests five common faults:

- incomplete literature searches
- only literature in English used
- failure to check the quality of papers to be included with due rigour
- poor analytical techniques
- conclusions that are not really supported by the results.[28]

With this in mind, a local prescribing committee may see the systematic review with meta-analysis as just what is required, but there will need to be a critical evaluation of the work to check it is of an acceptable standard.

Randomised controlled trials

The next tier down in the NICE hierarchy is evidence from one or more randomised controlled trials (RCTs). RCTs, of course, form the basis of the type of systematic review already discussed. An RCT is a method that seeks to investigate an intervention or course of action to establish the true effect. This is done by exposing one set of subjects to the intervention and having a similar set of subjects who are not exposed but, in every other way, are the same – the controls. The controls may well have a different intervention rather than nothing. Allocation to either set is undertaken in a truly random way. The subjects and those undertaking the research should be ignorant of the set to which specific individuals have been assigned, that is, the RCT is of a double-blind design. Ideally all those involved will be blinded – staff administering the intervention, taking measurements and so on.

A detailed discussion of trial design is beyond the scope of this book, but it is worth noting that not all RCTs are of the same quality; this section also examines some important aims and pitfalls. The care taken in trial design is to achieve validity – sometimes described as internal validity, to distinguish it from external validity – which, in turn, is also called generalisability. The latter was mentioned above in the context of pragmatic trials. Put simply, internal validity looks at whether the trial gives the right answer, whereas external validity looks at whether the trial gives a relevant answer.

Internal validity of a trial is undermined when bias arises; bias occurs where factors cause the study to overestimate or underestimate the true effect of the intervention. Bias can stem from several areas: selection of subjects, the way the intervention or general care is delivered, the way the effects are measured, the way withdrawals are handled, and the way the analysis is performed. Randomised entry, blinding, standardised care plans rigorously followed, and analysis on an intention-to-treat basis, are four key weapons in the battle against bias.

Confounding is another potential problem with studies, including with RCTs. Confounding occurs when the impact of the intervention is overestimated or underestimated because the trial result is altered by a factor other than the intervention. A confounding variable exists, which leads to the wrong conclusion. Typically such an error occurs if the control population is different from the intervention group in certain important ways not known to the investigator or the importance of which is not known. Confounding can also occur where an intervention being tested also requires some other aspect of care to change (more attention from the investigator perhaps); the positive effect demonstrated and attributed to the intervention could be caused by the other, unanalysed, change. Well-matched controls with equivalent care, other than the intervention, are used to eliminate confounding.

The section started with the idea that all RCTs are good, but has moved on to suggest that some are 'more good' than others. Having explained that bias and confounding can give 'the wrong answer', a third factor is that the trial result can mislead due to chance. As with trial design, a detailed discussion of hypothesis testing and of statistical analysis is beyond the scope of this book; here just a few concepts will be mentioned. *Pharmaceutical Statistics* by Jones provides a detailed discussion of these and other statistical matters and is aimed at pharmacists who may need to deal with these issues.[35] The purpose of using a statistical analysis in a trial is to explore if the conclusion is purely caused by chance; if the intervention is shown to be better than the control, it could really be better or, just because there will always be a spread of results, it may just seem better by chance, and if you repeated the same trial a further 10 times you may get the opposite answer every time.

To discuss significance, power and sample size, the null hypothesis is a good starting point. This is a statement that gives the essence of a trial, that the two courses of action explored give the same results. If the difference between one statin and another is to be explored, the null hypothesis might be: statin A and statin B have no difference in the percentage reduction of cholesterol after one year of standard daily dosing. Four scenarios could exist:

- The statins are equivalent and the trial shows that they are (the null hypothesis is supported).
- The statins are not equivalent and the trial shows that they are not equivalent (the null hypothesis is rejected – we can ignore for a moment whether A or B is better).
- The statins are truly equivalent but the trial shows that they are not (type 1 error – null hypothesis rejected when it was correct).
- The statins are truly not equivalent but the trial shows that they are (type 2 error – null hypothesis supported when it was false).

The probability of type 1 error is called the statistical significance level; the probability of type 2 error is called the power. Statistical significance or *p*-value therefore shows how likely it was the difference demonstrated in a trial was purely due to chance. Similarly, power is therefore the ability of a trial to show a difference when one really does exist. Conventionally, p-values of 5% are sought and power of 80% or better. Sample size helps address the uncertainty that chance brings. In essence, the larger the sample size, the more certain that a true answer has been reached (all else being equal). Thus a large trial of statin A versus statin B will have greater power than a small trial. Importantly, the sample size required to attain a given power will depend on the difference in effect expected and on the variability of the measure. Hardly surprisingly, large differences in effect are easier to detect than small ones.

It is worth noting that statistical significance has several problems. Statistical significance can be misinterpreted to mean clinical importance, when, as we have discussed, it is addressing the role of chance. For example, a very large, well-designed RCT might show statistically significant differences in cholesterol reduction between statin A and statin B, but a difference that in absolute terms is of no clinical importance whatsoever. The test for statistical significance is used to give a yes or no answer – if the p-value is below 5%, statistical significance is achieved. This is not as helpful to the reader as is the (now) more popular statement of confidence intervals.

The confidence interval is the range over which the result of a measurement in a trial is likely, with a specified level of certainty. Conventionally the 95% confidence interval is stated. Thus a figure is given (the answer) and then a range above and below that figure in which, 95 times out of 100, the real answer will lie. A large confidence interval shows the trial may be unhelpful; a trial where the 95% confidence intervals for two treatments overlap suggests they may in fact not truly differ. If treatments have truly large differences, even broad confidence intervals around the results will not overlap, whereas for truly small differences, a large sample size is required to produce tight confidence intervals. Figure 4.5 uses confidence intervals around the results of individual trials, presenting them as lines each side of a dot, but in figures they are typically presented in the form: n (95% CI $n - x$ to $n + x$) or, as an example, 3.4 (95% CI 3.1 to 3.7).

Statistical tests, methods of reviewing design and checking conclusions, are key tests in reviewing RCTs. As with systematic reviews, the medicines manager needs to be alert to potential flaws in the evidence.

Non-randomised and quasi-experimental studies

Levels IIa and IIb in the NICE hierarchy would be turned to when RCTs are not available. Non-randomised entry trials forego the benefits of randomised entry trials; they are, therefore, more prone to bias; the investigator could, for example, allocate those more likely to benefit to the intervention group. Level IIa evidence still requires controls, but not random allocation of subjects.

Quasi-experimental studies come in a variety of forms but usually take the intervention group and controls from a natural setting rather than established for the trial. As with non-randomised entry, risks of bias and of confounding exist. Attempts to match controls to the intervention group may be made.

Caution is required in the interpretation and use of level II evidence but decision making may still need to be informed by these methods.

The lower tiers

Level III in the NICE classification is evidence from non-experimental studies. Comparative studies, correlation studies and case studies are listed as possible sources of this descriptive work by NICE. For unusual therapies, uses outside the market authorisation, or for emerging therapies, this may be the only type of evidence available. If therapeutic committees are asked to review such uses regarding safety or cost, a degree of caution is required. Comparative studies include cohort studies and case control studies. Cohort studies look at a group of subjects over a period of time to identify events or changes; the results may then be compared with a control group. Thus, patients exposed to a specific medicine could be monitored over a five-year period to observe incidence of malignant disease, with the general population incidence used as a comparison. Case-control studies take a similar approach but look backwards to explore the cause of a disease or problem.

Case studies can also contribute information. They can be divided into case reports and case series; these are, respectively, single or a series of individual case histories. There are no attempts to control or blind, and confounding is a clear risk. They provide well-recorded, anecdotal evidence.

Level IV evidence is that of expert opinion, from respected bodies or individuals. In effect it is where the experience of clinicians is applied to a question. For therapeutic committees, this level of evidence cannot be ignored; indeed gathering it may be the opportunity to gain buy-in to the final decision. However, it should not be used to override evidence at higher levels in the hierarchy. For some decisions it may be all that is available.

Accessing the evidence

The various evidence types have been described. The emphasis has been on the use of systematic review of RCTs and on well-designed RCTs, with lower tiers of evidence used for questions of more unusual medicine use. How can these sources be accessed? Clearly, there are numerous journals with thousands of articles being published on a regular basis. Methods must be followed to access those that give good coverage – the right papers are found – without being too time consuming. There are now several electronic databases that allow medical and pharmaceutical and other journal articles to be searched, although there is no one source or database that covers all publications and there is also a time lag between publication and citation. Pharmacists who have worked in medicines information will have used the UKMi Training Workbook as an important training tool.[36] Section D of the Workbook deals with the basics of accessing information.[37] The web-based version is password-controlled for UKMi website users. MEDLINE is suggested as a key source for published papers. (MEDLINE is the accepted name for Medical Literature, Analysis and Retrieval System Online, an American database established in 1966. It can be accessed at www.ncbi.nlm.nih.gov and provides citations of biomedical literature, with or without abstracts, which may be searched using fairly simple techniques.) Access to MEDLINE may also be possible via local arrangements in NHS organisations, and support is available from most healthcare libraries.

EMBASE is another database and is available at www.embase.com or, again, for NHS organisations there may be locally arranged access. This has a broader coverage than MEDLINE, but it began more recently (1974).

For these, and the many other databases available, a structured approach to searching is required, relevant to the database and the question being pursued. Khan *et al.* neatly describe the approach as 'building a suitable combination of free text words and controlled terms' – the controlled terms being subject headings which are like tree branches with further subjects stemming from them as would twigs.[24] In this way the database is searched for all items where the chosen words or phrases appear. Restrictions, such as listing those where the word is in the title or as a key word, may be imposed. Restrictions on study design chosen and language used in publication are two further examples of limiting searches. Combining terms using Boolean logic allows the creation of limited sets of citations; the common terms are *and*, *or* and *not*, known as operators. Thus searching for 'bendrofluazide *and* hypertension' would list citations where both bendrofluazide and hypertension are included, whereas 'bendrofluazide *or* hypertension' provides a list of citations where bendrofluazide is mentioned, plus where hypertension is mentioned and includes all references where both are mentioned. As with any area of practice, skills need to be developed in this area and a good knowledge of the database used can avoid frustration.

Sources with important, but specific rather than broad, coverage include the *Cochrane Central Register of Controlled Trials* (CENTRAL) and a research register of ongoing trials found on the web at controlled-trials.com.

Although these search sites have been mentioned in the context of seeking primary sources and research studies, systematic reviews can also be found using the databases already mentioned. In addition, *The Cochrane Database of Systematic Reviews* can be used. Indeed this is an excellent first port of call in beginning a review of literature that is to be taken to a prescribing committee as it may mean a local review is not essential.

Whatever data are sought, the expertise of local medicines information staff and of librarians is an essential part of the process of accessing relevant papers. These staff have an important contribution to make in the successful delivery of strategic medicines management.

Finding systematic review and clinical trial reports is usually the first stage of the process of considering how a medicine should be used locally. However, there may be occasions when 'ready made' appraisals are available that need little extra work. The documents mentioned in the scanning and planning section may provide this. Documents from other health communities, such as the London New Drugs Group, may also provide relevant material. It may be that tailoring for local use takes a little work; the evidence base will be the same but local practice, experience and interests may be different. Although the cliché 'we don't want to re-invent the wheel' is often brought out when this subject is discussed, extending the metaphor used can remind us that considerable design work goes into getting the wheel just right for the latest Mercedes model.

Appraising the evidence

In describing the various evidence sources, potential weaknesses have been identified. Checking for these is an essential part of appraising the evidence to inform strategic medicines management decision making.

Critical appraisal of the evidence is an important way to combat pharmaceutical industry-led prescribing policy. Jones suggests the first question on examining a report is 'Is the trial sponsored?'[29] There may be a suspicion in many minds that the arrival, with media fanfare, of a new medicine is being stage managed by the manufacturer. Unquestioning acceptance of an abstract reporting an important new trial could be encouraged by such events.

Clark and Mucklow point out that appraising the evidence has two parts, assessing validity and checking clinical usefulness.[27] Their comments approximate to the questions:

- Is the evidence from trials that have internal validity?
- Is the evidence from trials that are generalisable?

More pertinently the second question could be stated: does the evidence apply to the circumstances we are considering? 'Circumstances' is used here as shorthand for all the relevant factors, including the population being treated, the disease, co-morbidity, dose and so on.

Appraising systematic reviews and meta-analyses

Greenhalgh published an introduction to these types of paper in the *British Medical Journal* in 1997.[38] She included a series of five questions that a reader of systematic reviews could use to review their quality. These form a helpful structure and other similar examples can be found in the literature; for example, Wiffen adapts a list from Oxman *et al.*[28] Greenhalgh's questions can be summarised as:

- Is there a clear question?
- Was there a thorough literature search? This should include a MEDLINE search, access to the Cochrane database, references cited in papers discovered in MEDLINE, access to 'grey' literature such as theses and government papers and should not restrict itself to English language. For emerging medicines, some of these sources are not likely to be relevant; for established therapeutic groups, they are.
- Was the methodology of the trials properly examined and did the summary give weight according to quality? The issues of internal validity, precision (dealing with chance) and external validity should have been addressed in the review.
- Would the conclusions have altered if the methodology had changed slightly? Greenhalgh suggests a sensitivity analysis of the review. Do the conclusions remain true if some minor changes are made? An example would be to re-examine the position if one of the less well-designed trials that favours the treatment is removed – if the treatment still appears effective, the review is robust.

- Have the numerical results been interpreted with common sense? The problem of confusing significance with importance, discussed earlier, comes into this question.

Khan *et al.* provide a much more detailed set of questions in their text on systematic reviews.[24] They include aspects such as whether review authors have stated clearly their criteria for including papers and whether the heterogeneity of the studies included has been assessed.

Where meta-analysis has been used, further questions should be raised. A key item is whether the data combined are truly combinable. This is an expansion of the heterogeneity question – is it reasonable to lump together patient populations, details of the intervention, the measures being combined and the settings of individual trials? Davies and Crombie also point to the dangers of inappropriate subgroup analysis.[34] By this, they mean taking subsets of trials and providing a summarised answer – exploration of data, not explanation, as they describe it.

A review of systematic reviews by Jadad *et al.*, concentrating on asthma treatment, is an important read for those using this type of evidence.[39] They examined 50 systematic reviews and meta-analyses and used Oxman and Guyatt's index as an assessment tool. (The Oxman and Guyatt index can be found in the *Journal of Clinical Epidemiology* 1991; 44: 1271–1278.) They found that 40 of the 50 reviews were seriously or extensively flawed. They noted that of the 10 better papers, seven were found in the *Cochrane Library* and that those reviews funded by industry were usually flawed; these flaws meant the reviews were poor as a guide to decision making. Jadad *et al.* do point out that the tool used to assess quality was developed by Andrew Oxman, who was also key in developing the Cochrane methodology. The underlying rule then is to remain cautious and critical of evidence, even from published systematic reviews.

Appraising randomised controlled trials

In describing systematic reviews earlier in the chapter, there was some mention of appraising RCTs, because that is what systematic reviews do. Here a few specific issues and sources of assessment tools will be mentioned.

Greenhalgh's series of articles in the *British Medical Journal* in 1997, later published as a text, provided a number of helpful papers on assessing articles, including the item on reviews described earlier and items on methodology and on statistics.[38,40–42] Clark and Mucklow set out a checklist for appraising a therapy article. It includes asking if the authors are respected in the field, through to the strengths of the statistical tests.[27] Clearly, putting too much weight on the former question would be unwise – good authors can write bad books. Wiffen provides a list based on work by Guyatt, Sackett and Cook.[28] His questions address the following issues:

- Was the question clear?
- Was entry truly random?
- Did the analysis include all the subjects and was it analysed as assigned? ['Intention to treat' analysis is implied here.]
- Was there blinding of subjects, investigators and all involved?
- Was the control group appropriately matched to the intervention group?
- Was the control group treated in the same way as subjects other than the specified intervention?
- How large was the treatment effect? Was there clinical significance?
- How precise was the estimate of the treatment effect? Was there statistical significance? Was an appropriate statistical test used? Was statistical advice sought?
- Are the results generalisable and applicable to the local population in particular? Were inappropriately strict inclusion/exclusion criteria used?
- Were all clinically important outcomes considered? For example, in an antiplatelet therapy study, the bleeds as well as the protection ought to be considered.
- Are the gains from the intervention worth the harms and costs? This deals more with applying results than the quality of the study, unless an economic analysis is included.

Issues of sponsorship and authors' interests, whether the article was peer reviewed and the quality of the journal are in some ways relevant, but more in terms of raising a caution than actually altering the quality of the paper under consideration.

Presenting the evidence

Finding and appraising the evidence has a purpose, to inform the decision-making process on the managed entry of new medicines and controlled access of established products. Chapter 6 looks at using evidence for the additional purpose of preparing guidelines. How should evidence be presented for decision making? There is not one right way to present evidence regarding medicines – it will depend on the audience and the nature of the process being followed. A few of the issues will be discussed here.

There are four key questions that a presentation to a therapeutic committee should address:

- What is the question being examined?
- What process has been followed?
- What has been found?
- What conclusion does this suggest?

What is the question being examined?

This is a fairly obvious starting point, but in work carried out for therapeutic committees it is easily overlooked. Those undertaking critical appraisal should ensure that their brief is mutually understood before a significant piece of work is undertaken. An example of potential confusion would be as follows: the formulary pharmacist is asked whether atorvastatin or simvastatin should be first line on the coronary care unit, a literature search is undertaken, a useful systematic review is found and that, with some more recent papers, is summarised and presented; at the committee, a debate arises about starting dose (this had not been fully examined), the chief pharmacist then points out that the system would be much easier if there were to be one first-line statin across the trust, not just post-infarct: frustration ensues. Even well-planned questions may result in a concern that knowing just one or two more things could give a better decision, but some pragmatism will always be required. Given a clear brief and having completed the task, the decision makers should be given a clear statement of what is and is not addressed by the appraisal.

What process has been followed?

An explanation of what literature searching was undertaken, by whom and what appraisal or synthesis followed, should be stated. If all that was done was to seek an NPC/UKMi document or a London New Drugs Group monograph, then that should be made clear. Any consultation with local experts should be reported; it may be helpful to include them in the process, as they will inevitably be affected by the decision made.

What has been found?

This covers two issues: what documents were available and what did they say? The sources used for the appraisal should be stated, a comment on the quality of the reviews or trials used made, then a statement of the benefits or outcomes or effects that are relevant to the question

Table 4.4 Number needed to treat (NNT)

	Number treated in trial	Number responding	NNT
Treatment A	350	35	10
Treatment B	360	40	9

When considering a move from A to B, how many subjects need to be switched for there to be one extra responder? This gives a further NNT. The NNT for the switch is 100.

posed. Members of the decision-making group may wish to have access to the papers directly, rather than relying on an appraiser, but it is unlikely that all members of therapeutic and prescribing committees will have time to study all papers themselves.

Summarising the evidence into a single measure may not always be appropriate, but it often can play a part in decision making. When doing this it is important not to drift into the realm of 'pseudo-marketing', where the best-possible sounding summary may be presented. To give an example: if the standard medicine has an incidence of a side-effect at 0.5% and the new medicine has an incidence of 0.4%, it would be true to say there is a 20% reduction in the incidence of the side-effect, but stating this relative change without the absolute figures could mislead. The term 'absolute risk reduction' is used to describe the actual difference in the rate of a particular event in the intervention group compared with the control. From this figure a useful and increasingly popular summary measure can be derived: the numbers needed to treat (NNT). Most simply put, the NNT is the number of subjects you need to treat for one of them to benefit. The timeframe should also be stated. Thus if a treatment cures 5% of patients treated, the NNT is 20. In comparing two treatments, a simple proportion calculation is required. Table 4.4 gives a fictitious example. Similarly a summary of numbers needed to harm (NNH) could be stated; thus, for aspirin in secondary prevention of stroke, an NNT could be stated and an NNH comparison could be made with other anti-platelet medicines.

Chapter 5 discusses health economic issues, but if health economic data are available, or even just costings, these will be required by decision makers in many circumstances, although as discussed in Chapter 2, arrangements for committee structures do vary across organisations.

What does the evidence suggest?

A simple, clearly presented conclusion will usually be welcomed by the decision-making group. However, this must be supported by the evidence and must be cautious if the evidence is weak. It may be that matters of affordability and relative benefits (compared with all other developments) must be considered alongside the evidence presented, but a well-presented conclusion or evidence summary should help this. Local committees will have their own preferences for how this is done and conclusions need to suit the question asked, but there should be some indication of the strength of evidence and some indication of the 'direction' of the answer. An example (although things are rarely as simple) could be: there was little evidence found to show a difference in effectiveness between analgesic A and the current formulary choice; analgesic A caused less constipation in chronic use but this has little relevance to the proposed postoperative role; analgesic A is considerably more expensive.

Coming to a decision

The process of gathering, assessing and presenting the evidence has been described. The emphasis has been on effectiveness. Chapter 5 concentrates on the economic considerations and Chapter 8 considers budgetary matters. However, these aspects are mentioned here as they are vital to decision making. The hurdles of efficacy, effectiveness, costs and benefits, and affordability, are central to the decision-making process for new medicine entry and for looking at classes of established medicines. Efficacy, it was argued, is dealt with by licensing. For situations outside the market authorisation, or for unlicensed medicines, appraisal of the (probably) limited evidence may help. These uses will probably be more related to individuals rather than part of strategic medicines management, but this is not always so. In such situations the efficacy question merges with the effectiveness one, where the process of examining evidence described earlier is followed.

Decision making will require judgements to be made. These may be supported by considerable or by scanty data. In deciding whether to support access to a new medicine, the decision-making group will need to examine not only whether there is any evidence of additional benefits and reduced risks, but also whether the medicine is likely to be preferred by patients because of ease of administration or that the regimen is easier to follow. These advantages will then need to be weighed against the additional costs, and if there are several items competing for the same costs, how the benefits of the proposed change compares with others. Some pragmatism may be required in reaching a decision. Imposing strong restrictions that will be ignored or fought against by prescribers may not be worthwhile if a compromise can be reached imposing some control that will gain adherence.

Conclusion

Making decisions about access to new medicines and the use of established ones requires an examination and understanding of the evidence. Local organisations need access to reasonably rapid, high-quality critical appraisal of the evidence. Critical-appraisal skills may be available locally in medicines information centres and among PCT pharmacists. Although evidence review is a time-consuming process, it is important if advert-led prescribing is to be avoided. Summarising the evidence and bringing in issues of 'bang for buck' and affordability will need to be undertaken at a therapeutic or prescribing committee level. This should be done across a health community and, where possible, by developing a pragmatic consensus. The detail of how this is done will depend on local circumstances.

References

1. The Medicines and Healthcare Regulatory Authority. Medicines section. http://medicines.mhra.gov.uk (accessed 8 December 2004).
2. British Medical Association and the Royal Pharmaceutical Society. *British National Formulary*, 46th edn, London: BMA and RPS, 2003.
3. British Medical Association and the Royal Pharmaceutical Society. *British National Formulary*, 47th edn, London: BMA and RPS, 2004.
4. Grattini S, Bertele V. Efficacy, safety, and cost of new anticancer drugs. *Br Med J* 2002; 325: 269–271.
5. Ma J, Stafford R, Cockburn I, Finkelstein S. A statistical analysis of the magnitude and composition of drug promotion in the United States in 1998. *Clin Ther* 2003; 25: 1503–1517.
6. Moynihon R. Who pays for the pizza? Redefining the relationships between doctors and drug companies. 1: Entanglement. *Br Med J* 2003; 236: 1189–1192.
7. Wolfe S. Drug advertisements that go straight to the hippocampus. *Lancet* 1996; 348: 632.
8. Kessler D. Addressing the problem of misleading advertising. *Ann Intern Med* 1992; 116: 950–951.
9. Calfee J. The role of marketing in pharmaceutical research and development. *Pharmacoeconomics* 2002; 20 (S, 3): 72–85.
10. Tucker G. Science and drug therapy: ins and outs, ups and downs. *Pharm J* 1995; 255: 376–379.
11. Temple R, Himmel M. Safety of newly approved drugs: implications for prescribing. *JAMA* 2002; 287: 2273–2275.

12. Lasser K, Allen P, Woolhandler S. *et al.* Timing of blackbox warnings and withdrawals for prescription medications. *JAMA* 2002; 287: 2215–2220.

13. Efexor safety message, MHRA website. http://medicines.mhra.gov.uk/ourwork/monitorsafequalmed/safetymessages/efexor0903.pdf (accessed 8 December 2004).

14. Department of Health. *Building a Safer NHS for Patients: Improving Medication Safety.* London: DH, 2004.

15. Department of Health. Chapter 11, sections 11 and 12. *The NHS Plan: A Plan for Investment, a Plan for Reform.* Norwich: The Stationery Office, 2000.

16. Harman R. The drug development process: 1 Introduction and overview. *Pharm J* 1999; 262: 234–237.

17. Brzezicki A. Responding to new developments – the challenge for PCTs. *Future Prescriber* 2004; 5: 3.

18. Golightly P. Medicines information. In Stephens M, ed. *Hospital Pharmacy.* London: Pharmaceutical Press, 2003.

19. Horizon Scanning Centre, Birmingham. http://www.publichealth.bham.ac.uk/horizon/partnerships1.htm (accessed 8 December 2004).

20. Horizon Scanning Centre, Birmingham. 90Y-muHMFG1 (R1549) for ovarian cancer (July 2003). http://pcpoh.bham.ac.uk/publichealth/horizon/cancer.htm (accessed 15 December 2004).

21. National Prescribing Centre. New drugs. http://www.npc.co.uk/new_drugs.htm (accessed 8 December 2004).

22. Davis H (Executive editor). *Prescribing Outlook – August 2003 Part A.* UKMi and NPC, 2003.

23. Sennik D, Erskine D. *Prescribing Outlook – October 2003 Part B.* London: UKMi, 2003.

24. Khan K, Kunz R, Kleinjnen J, Antes G. *Systematic Reviews to Support Evidence-Based Medicine.* London: Royal Society of Medicine Press, 2003.

25. Sackett D, Rosenberg W, Gray J. *et al.* Evidence-based medicine: what it is and isn't. *Br Med J* 1996; 312: 71–72.

26. Jones C. Evidence-based medicine: (1) research methods. *Pharm J* 2002; 268: 839–841.

27. Clark W, Mucklow J. Gathering and weighing the evidence. In Panton R, Chapman S, eds. *Medicines Management.* London: BMJ Publishing Group and Pharmaceutical Press 1998.

28. Wiffen P. *Evidence-based Pharmacy.* Oxford: Radcliffe Medical Press, 2001.

29. Jones C. Evidence based medicine: (2) how to appraise a clinical paper. *Pharm J* 2002; 268: 875–877.

30. Jones C. Evidence based medicine: (3) where to find evidence. *Pharm J* 2002; 269: 677–679.

31. Moore A, McQuay H. Type and strength of efficacy evidence. *Bandolier* 1997; 4: 8.

32. Antithrombotic Trialists' Collaboration. Collaborative meta-analysis of randomised trials of antiplatelet therapy for prevention of death, myocardial infarction and stroke in high risk patients. *Br Med J* 2002; 324: 71–86.

33. Furukawa T, McGuire H, Barbui C. Meta-analysis of effects and side effects of low dosage tricyclic antidepressants in depression: systematic review. *Br Med J* 2002; 325: 991–999.

34. Davies H, Crombie I. What is meta-analysis? 2004; 1(8): 1–9. http://www.evidence-based-medicine.co.uk/ebmfiles/WhatisMetaAn.pdf (accessed 28 February 2005).

35. Jones D. *Pharmaceutical Statistics*. London: Pharmaceutical Press, 2002.

36. UKMi Workbook. http://www.ukmi.nhs.uk/secure/training/workbook/default.asp (Registration required; accessed 1 April 2004).

37. UKMi Workbook. http://www.ukmi.nhs.uk/secure/training/workbook/pdfs/IntroductionSectionD.pdf (Registration required; accessed 1 April 2004).

38. Greenhalgh T. How to read a paper: papers that summarise other papers (systematic reviews and meta-analyses). *Br Med J* 1997; 315: 672–675.

39. Jadad A, Moher M, Browman G. *et al.* Systematic reviews and meta-analyses on treatments of asthma: critical evaluation. *Br Med J* 2000; 320: 537–540.

40. Greenhalgh T. How to read a paper: assessing the methodological quality of a published paper. *Br Med J* 1997; 315: 305–308.

41. Greenhalgh T. How to read a paper: statistics for the non statistician: significant relations and their pitfalls. *Br Med J* 1997; 315: 422–425.

42. Greenhalgh T. *How to Read a Paper: the Basics of Evidence-Based Medicine*. London: BMJ Publishing Group, 1997.

5

Health economics

Lord Robbins described economics as 'the science which studies human behaviour as a relationship between ends and scarce means, which have alternative uses'.[1] Packed into this sentence are two of the fundamentals of economics: scarcity and opportunity cost. 'Scarcity' is the principle that there are not sufficient resources to do everything you might wish to do; 'opportunity cost' refers to the fact that if you use your resources for one thing, you have to do without something else. The opportunity cost is sometimes described as the benefits foregone by taking one course of action rather than another. More recently than Lord Robbins, Samuelson described economics as 'the way society ends up choosing'.[2] This could be understood as the ways and means by which it is decided which benefits are chosen and which are foregone. Such decisions are a key part of strategic medicines management.

Economics can be divided into macroeconomics and microeconomics. Macroeconomics deals with whole systems, the issues affecting the nation; microeconomics deals with the economics of 'the firm' or of specific elements. Health economics is the application of microeconomics to the field of healthcare. The term pharmacoeconomics, often used in pharmacy literature, is the application of health economics to medicines.

Health economics provides a conceptual framework and a set of techniques or tools that can assist the decision maker. Chapter 4 explains how information on effectiveness can be found, assessed and presented; it acknowledges that a judgement is needed to determine how extra costs may be traded off for increased safety or for extra benefits. This is where health economics can assist, although the need for judgement to be applied will remain.

In this chapter, a short discussion of some of the concepts of health economics is followed by a description of the analytical techniques; a guide to assessing the quality of health economic papers is given and examples of health economics used in the context of medicines concludes the chapter.

Economic concepts

Health economics considers interventions in terms of inputs and outputs. Inputs are the resources used for the intervention – the costs – outputs are the effects, taken broadly, of the intervention – the benefits. Economic analyses examine inputs and outputs of two or more courses of action, one of which could be the 'do nothing' option. The different types of analysis will be explored later. In the context of strategic medicines management, the inputs will often be the costs associated with providing a medicine, not just the acquisition costs of the product, and the outputs, the health gain and associated benefits.

Cost-effectiveness is a term used loosely to mean 'economically worthwhile'.[3] In economics it has a specific meaning in the context of analyses, but it also implies an aspect of efficiency. Efficiency also has usage in physics and engineering: it is the way of comparing systems in terms of their production of outputs from given inputs. As an example, a newly designed light-bulb is said to have increased efficiency compared with the standard if it can produce the same amount of light using less electricity. Economists use the term 'efficiency' in a similar way. Efficiency is said to increase if there are more outputs from the same inputs or the same output from less input. However, health economists have divided efficiency into two terms: 'technical efficiency' and 'allocative efficiency'.

Technical efficiency looks at an intervention and compares the output:input ratio, just as with the light-bulb. An example more relevant to medicines would be that technical efficiency is increased if a switch is made from a premium-branded product to an equivalent generic product – so long as the benefits from treatment remained unaltered. This is a simple illustration – technical efficiency can be increased even when benefits change, the key issue being whether the ratio of what you get out compared with what you put in improves.

Allocative efficiency looks at the bigger picture. It means considering how the whole package of possible inputs is used to produce outputs and whether, by changing what we do, a greater level of output could be achieved. Allocative efficiency is where we seek to use resources in a way that maximises benefits. Donaldson and Gerard described this as pursuing programmes where health benefits outweigh the costs and, by implication, not undertaking health interventions where costs outweigh benefits.[4] For strategic medicines management, increasing allocative efficiency could include taking a decision to invest in statins to prevent stroke rather than in a high-cost, new cancer therapy that

Box 5.1 Average and marginal costs.

Costs for treating 10 patients = £100
Costs for treating 11 patients = £101
Average costs for treating 10 patients = £100 ÷ 10 = £10
Average costs for treating 11 patients = £101 ÷ 11 = £9.18
Marginal cost of treating 11th patient = £101 − £100 = £1

only gave a very small health gain. Such decisions are difficult, but allocative efficiency acknowledges that resources are finite and that choices must be made. The aim is to choose interventions that maximise health gains from the limited resources available.

Another idea that is of importance in economics is the margin. When considering a change in the way resources are used, switching from one medicine to another, perhaps, it is the difference caused by the change that is particularly important. This is a fairly obvious statement but is an idea sometimes overlooked in analyses. The concept of the margin describes this difference. The marginal benefit from a new medicine compared with an old one is the extra lives saved, cures achieved, or improved quality of life from the new product. Likewise, the marginal costs of a treatment are the extra costs of a new treatment compared with the old, or the costs of treating the extra patient(s) if a programme is expanded. The marginal cost is thus differentiated from the average cost; the average cost being the total cost of an activity divided by the volume of that activity. Box 5.1 works through an example of costs stated at the margin and as average. In some circumstances these differences will not be important, but there are circumstances where using the average rather than the margin can mislead. Box 5.2 gives two examples of such cases. Example A shows that, although the average cost of a more effective prophylactic regimen remains attractive compared with the cost of treating the disease, at the margin, the five additional cases prevented by the better regimen are in fact prevented at five times the cost of treatment. This is, of course, a very simplistic example, with the assumption that there are no disbenefits in treating the disease. Example B explores the reasonable cut-off point for a particular aspect of a hypothetical secondary prevention of a myocardial infarct. Looking at the average treatment cost per infarct avoided, even the extended therapy may seem attractive – although at a glance it can be seen that no extra gains are made after nine months.

Box 5.2 When average and marginal costs matter.

Example A
Alternative prophylactic regimens exist for a disease. The costs and effectiveness are shown as:

- Regimen I prevents disease in 90% of cases and costs £10 per patient.
- Regimen II prevents disease in 95% of cases and costs £15 per patient.

Treatment of the disease where prophylaxis fails is £20.

Considering the average cost per case avoided:

- Regimen I has a cost-effectiveness ratio of £11.11 per case avoided.
- Regimen II has a cost-effectiveness ratio of £15.80 per case avoided.

(These are derived from calculating total spend divided by number of cases avoided, e.g. for regimen I: 100 × £10 divided by 90 cases.)

Thus the *average* cost for each regimen is less than the cost of treatment.

Considering the marginal extra costs of regimen II compared with regimen I: Assume a population of 100 patients. Cost of using regimen I is £1000 for prophylaxis but 10 cases will need treatment. Cost of using regimen II is £1500 but five cases will require treatment.

Therefore £500 is spent avoiding five cases. The marginal cost per extra case avoided is £100. This is much greater than the cost of treating a case.

Example B
A hypothetical treatment to avoid a recurrence of myocardial infarct (MI)

Months of treatment	0	3	6	9	12
MI avoided	0	12	15	16	16
Costs per 100 patients (£)	0	6000	12000	18000	24000
Average cost per MI avoided (£)	NA	500	800	1125	1500
Stepped marginal cost (£)	NA	500	2000	6000	No extra MIs avoided

The stepped marginal cost is derived by looking at the extra costs and extra MIs avoided compared with the previous column, e.g. for the six-month column: three extra cases are avoided compared with three months but an extra £6000 is incurred, so stepped marginal cost is £6000 divided by three cases avoided = £2000 per case avoided.

The marginal analysis gives a much clearer picture and is more helpful for the cut-off point decision. This is an important issue when reviewing pharmacoeconomic cases and articles.

Example B in Box 5.2 also provides an example of another concept in economics – diminishing marginal utility. The essence of this is that the benefit gained from the, say, 10th good purchased is likely to be a little less than that gained from the ninth and so on. To put into an everyday context: the pleasure gained from consuming our fifth bar of chocolate at one sitting is probably less than eating the first one. There are of course clear exceptions, but generally the rule applies to some degree. In the health context, extending therapies from those who gain biggest benefits to those who gain some benefit often happens as access to treatments is broadened. In the example in Box 5.2, the marginal gains by extending treatment from three to six months is three events avoided; the gain for the next three-month extension is just one event avoided. The same pattern can emerge when adding further medicines to a regimen – extra benefits may be gained at less attractive ratios of cost to benefit. The first medicine gives the easy win, the second saves a few more lives in the population, the third helps a little and so on. Additionally, issues of adherence to regimens, even if the patient wishes to take all the items, may fall away. Thus it is actually harder to get the extra benefits from the fourth and fifth medicine, because patients get muddled or forgetful (in some cases).

The goal of increased efficiency and the importance of the margin are vital features of health economics. A further issue, sometimes overlooked, is equity. The Department of Health documents *New NHS Modern Dependable* and *Saving Lives: Our Healthier Nation* both mention the concept of equity.[5,6] The former talks of seeking 'no more post code prescribing', the latter of prioritising the improvements in health of those worst off in society. These illustrate two themes of equity: people with equivalent needs should have them met, whatever their circumstances (sometimes called horizontal equity); those with greater needs require greater help (sometimes called vertical equity). This is a very large subject, but a key point for note here is that seeking equity means that healthcare decisions are not just about maximising health benefits but also about distributive justice tempering the goal of efficiency. Bringing equity into prescribing committee decisions may be harder than concentrating on health benefits but it has great relevance. An example would be where capping the number of patients who can receive a high-cost medicine is considered; to do so arbitrarily is inequitable. Drawing a line to limit therapy to those most likely to benefit or those with greatest need could be considered equitable, even if this proves difficult or exposes the health community to financial risk.

Some of the basic concepts of health economics have been outlined so far – more detailed discussion can readily been found in texts by Drummond, Mooney and others, and an NPC bulletin was issued in 2000 that provides a brief introduction.[4,7,8]

Economic analyses

Health economic analyses compare alternative treatments or interventions in terms of their inputs and outputs. Three techniques are, conventionally, distinguished; each technique measures inputs in terms of financial costs but vary in how outputs are measured. Table 5.1 gives a simple summary of these three basic techniques, plus two other methods that are a variation on these. Each of the three will be explored in more detail and their application to strategic medicines management considered.

Cost-effectiveness analysis

Cost-effectiveness analysis (CEA) is probably the most straightforward of the three techniques. CEA examines an intervention or course of action in comparison with another or with a do-nothing option. Costs and effects are considered. The result is a ratio of costs to effects stated for each alternative. In CEA the effects are restricted to a unidimensional output, stated in a simple naturalistic unit. Examples of such outputs are deaths avoided, ulcers healed, infections prevented.

CEA may be useful to compare interventions that seek to provide the same output. CEA certainly helps answer the question: 'Which of these two antibiotics is a better choice, in terms of efficiency, for prophylaxis?' in a specific perioperative situation. However, CEA begins to be less helpful where there are a number of different side-effects or complications. A choice may be presented: treatment A comes at £100 per ulcer healed but can give prolonged periods of nausea; treatment B comes at £105 per ulcer healed but can occasionally cause very severe headache. A is more cost-effective than B, and even allowing for treatments for nausea and headache, may remain so, but the CEA only takes us so far. CEA is even less helpful where choices between very different therapies are required and cannot contribute to the wider allocative efficiency debate. Comparing the gains from myocardial infarct prevention with those of slowing the onset of dementia cannot be addressed using CEA. This is where the next technique comes in.

Table 5.1 Health economic analyses

Name	Summary	How inputs measured	How ouputs measured
Cost-effectiveness analysis (CEA)	Means of comparing two or more interventions where outputs can be measured in the same way	£	A simple, natural unit, e.g. lives saved, cures, events avoided
Cost-utility analysis (CUA)	Means of comparing interventions that can be of very different types by creating a common 'currency' of output	£	Health gain, using a constructed index such as QALY or HYE
Cost–benefit analysis (CBA)	Means of comparing interventions of any kind and of exploring whether an intervention has a net cost or a net benefit	£	£
Cost-consequence analysis	Not formally a type of analysis but can be useful in comparing interventions that a pure CEA (using one measure) cannot address	£	As for CEA but several simple measures stated
Cost-minimisation analysis	CEA where the effects (outputs) are equivalent or assumed to be equivalent	£	Assumed equal

QALY = quality-adjusted life year; HYE = healthy years equivalent.

Cost–utility analysis

Cost–utility analysis (CUA) is similar to CEA, but replaces the natural-istic output measure with a constructed unit. Often, CEA is now used broadly to cover analyses that fit the CUA definition to be described here. Gray and Vale do not distinguish between CEA using simple output measures and CUA using constructed indices.[9] Here I hope the distinction does assist with clarity.

The concept of 'utility' appears frequently in economics; it can be explained as the amount of satisfaction an individual gains from a good or service. CUA is a tool that seeks to compare dissimilar interventions by converting outputs into a measure of health gain. Rather than, as in CEA, examining a single effect of treatment, CUA seeks to combine two or more key factors of health into a single measure. Once achieved, a ratio of cost to this measure can be stated. The most commonly used measure is the quality-adjusted life year (QALY). CUA produces state-ments such as: intervention A costs £10,000 per QALY gained whereas intervention B costs £20,000 per QALY.

Alan Williams of York University published a *British Medical Journal* paper using CUA in 1985 in which the QALY was used as an output measure.[10] His stated aim was to allow comparison of coronary artery bypass grafting with other 'claimants on resources of the NHS'. CUA continues to be a potential source of help for such questions.

A QALY is a unit combining extension of life with a crude measure of health-related quality of that life. The two factors are multiplied together to result in the QALY outcome. The 'quality of life' is stated as a value on a scale where 1 is perfect health and 0 is equivalent to death. Thus where a treatment gives three extra years of life, but the health-related quality score is 0.8, then the output of the treatment is 2.4 QALY. Figure 5.1 gives an illustration of this, where the intervention both extends and improves quality.

An obvious question is, how are the scores for health-related quality of life derived? Kind, Rosser and Williams developed a scoring system using two a dimensional model – distress and disability.[11] They asked a group of subjects to score various hypothetical health states on the 0–1 scale. Most states fell into the 0.9 to 1 range, but some states scored less than 0, meaning that the respondents felt their health state was worse than being dead. Table 5.2 gives the possible options with scores. Even where the health state was such that there was severe distress and social restrictions the 'utility' of life was over 90% of perfect health.

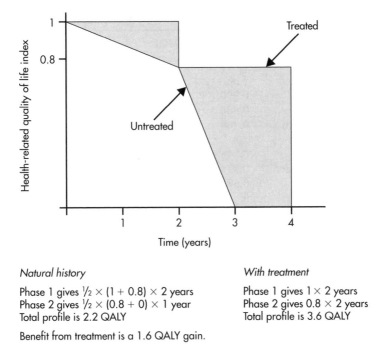

Natural history

Phase 1 gives $\frac{1}{2} \times (1 + 0.8) \times 2$ years
Phase 2 gives $\frac{1}{2} \times (0.8 + 0) \times 1$ year
Total profile is 2.2 QALY

Benefit from treatment is a 1.6 QALY gain.

With treatment

Phase 1 gives 1×2 years
Phase 2 gives 0.8×2 years
Total profile is 3.6 QALY

Figure 5.1 The quality-adjusted life year (QALY) gain (shaded area) from an intervention. In this case the natural history of disease survival is three years but with a falling, health-related quality of life. With treatment, survival is four years and with a retained quality of life.

The Kind–Rosser–Williams index described above has now been superseded by the scoring system derived from the EuroQol Group's EQ-5D instrument.[12] This a validated instrument that gives an evaluation of a health state by rating each of five dimensions at one of three levels. The dimensions are: mobility, self-care, usual activities, pain/discomfort, anxiety/depression. Scores of 1 for each (1,1,1,1,1) would mean a health state with no problems in walking, self-care or undertaking normal activities and where no pain, discomfort, anxiety or depression was present. Scores of 3 for each (3,3,3,3,3) would mean the person was bedridden, unable to do much at all, suffering severe pain or discomfort, and extremely anxious or depressed. A possible 243 health states exist in this system. These 'five figure' results have been converted into single scores, used in the same way that the Kind–Rosser–Williams index figures are. (McCulloch gives a good summary of deriving the EQ-5D coefficients in *Valuing Health in Practice*, Ashgate, 2003.) The scores have

Table 5.2 Kind, Rosser and Williams health state matrix

Disability	No distress	Mild distress	Moderate distress	Severe distress
None	1.00	0.995	0.990	0.967
Slight social	0.990	0.986	0.973	0.932
Severe social	0.980	0.972	0.956	0.912
Work and social functions affected	0.964	0.956	0.942	0.870
No paid work	0.946	0.935	0.900	0.700
Wheelchair confinement	0.875	0.845	0.860	0
Bed bound	0.677	0.564	0	–0.49
Unconscious	0	NA	NA	NA

NA = not applicable.

been reported based on a UK survey by Dolin et al.[13] The gain from a treatment can be evaluated as the extra years of life multiplied by the EuroQol-derived score of the health state of that life.

There are other methods of deriving QALY gains of health interventions. These are probably closer to economic theory than the two methods described, but less accessible. Each deals with hypothetical choices. The time trade-off approach explores how many years a person would give up if they could be in perfect health, rather than continue in their state of ill health. The person trade-off explores a similar issue but by asking which of two groups would the respondent restore to full health; the groups would have different health states and you would vary the numbers in each. The standard gamble explores the odds of dying that you would be prepared to accept to risk a treatment that could restore you from a given state of ill health to full health. Although mentioned for completeness, these techniques probably will not have great relevance to those engaged in strategic medicines management.

The QALY is not presented as a perfect measure and has had many critics. Earl-Slater and Norwood summarise the concerns in their discussion of health economics and drug use:[14]

- Is it reasonable to compare QALY over time and across different groups?
- QALY favours the young as intervening to save their lives has a long stream of gain compared with saving the lives of the old
- Is it only the patient's value of their health state that matters?
- The health-related quality of life score depends on the method used, so comparing different studies may be inappropriate.

On the fourth point Brazier *et al.* point out that published CUA often fail to state how their health state measures were derived, making comparison difficult.[15] Williams' paper used the Kind–Rosser–Williams index and had expert opinions to value the different health states.[10]

NICE technology appraisals report CUA that are available for the question under consideration, for example, appraisal 55 quotes an analysis where the incremental cost per QALY of paclitaxel combined with platinum therapy compared with carboplatin alone was £5273.[16] NICE does point out that, in that particular case, caution in interpretation is required. The literature has many examples of CUA and the use of these by pharmaceutical companies as well as by NICE is likely to lead to their increased appearance.

For the strategic medicines management decision maker, CUA gives an opportunity, albeit fraught with weaknesses, of comparing different medicines in terms of their ability to provide health gains. With a development fund of £50,000 to spend, the cost per QALY rating of five possible options could inform the decision-making process.

Cost–benefit analysis

Cost–benefit analysis (CBA) has been described as the most comprehensive method of health economic evaluation.[17] It seeks to value all outputs and inputs in monetary terms. CUA concentrates on health gain, CBA seeks to examine benefits including, but limited to, health gain. CBA, because it turns outputs into a monetary value, can also explore the question: 'Do the benefits of this intervention outweigh the costs?' CEA and CUA tell you what you get for your money, CBA tells you if you have gained more than you spent. Like CUA, CBA can also compare very different interventions and allow examination of the outputs of each.

Although a powerful tool, CBA has a difficulty – how can you convert the health gain, and other benefits, into a financial value? Willingness to pay is a methodology used to address this issue.[18,19] The financial value of the intervention is assessed by asking people what they would be willing to pay to make the gains. This is done by asking people with specific experience of the health state or by asking the general public. However, there are two major concerns – stated willingness to pay is almost certainly influenced by ability to pay (even in hypothetical situations) and whether the right people are being asked to provide the answers. Donaldson and Shackley provide a helpful discussion of willingness to pay with examples of its use, in their chapter in *Advances in Health Economics*.[20]

CBA will be particularly helpful where medicines have benefits beyond health gain. Thus, treatments for Alzheimer's disease, where social care costs are a big factor, would be better assessed using CBA, than addressing the health gain in terms of cost per QALY. Although this technique may be the most comprehensive, in practice it will not often be available as published evidence for the strategic medicines management decision maker.

Critical appraisal of economic analyses

Just as systematic reviews and clinical trials vary in quality, so do economic analyses. Various checklists have been suggested; Wiffen adapts the Drummond *et al.* checklist from their *Methods for Economic Evaluation of Health Care Programmes*.[21,22] Haycox and Walley also provided a series of questions which will be covered briefly here.[23]

Is the question appropriate and asked in an appropriate way?

There needs to be a clear statement in the analysis of what is being examined and what are the comparators. If being used by a therapeutic or prescribing committee, the question posed needs to be applicable to the question under consideration.

What is the perspective of the study?

An important consideration in economic analysis is the perspective taken. This was mentioned earlier in the context of willingness to pay methodology – there it was noted that differences in valuation may arise between the sufferer and the general public; this raises the question: 'Whose valuation should we take?' This is one aspect of the perspective issue. More broadly the whole costs and benefits question can be taken from different standpoints. Health economists would usually expect a societal perspective to be taken, that is, the way costs and benefits are assessed should include everything, not just those that fall on the NHS or on the patient. However, it may be that a prescribing committee wishes to be guided in its decision making only by NHS costs. Therefore using CUA, where health gain and a limited perspective of costs are taken, may be the most appropriate tool. A danger is that interventions where impact on social care is an important factor, such as treatment for Alzheimer's disease, will not get such a favourable hearing compared with an intervention that has all its benefits in the NHS/health arena.

Is the technique appropriate?

CEA, CUA and CBA each deal with outputs differently. The appropriate technique will depend on the intervention being examined and the question posed. The paper being reviewed should state clearly which technique was employed and it should be fit for purpose for the prescribing committee. CEA may be adequate for a choice between therapies for a specific disease, but CUA or CBA will be required if there is a need to prioritise a list of potential developments.

Is the comparator appropriate?

As with clinical trials, economic analyses should compare the new agent with the accepted best standard treatment.

Is the economic analysis supported by good clinical evidence?

The comments made in Chapter 4 about the quality of trial evidence apply equally to economic analyses. Poorly designed trials open to bias and confounding will result in misleading economic analyses.

There is an additional comment regarding trial evidence: basing costs on a clinical trial may lead to 'inflation' caused by protocol-driven costs such as extra visits or extra tests. Having said that, there may also be an overstatement of benefits owing to better concordance or the trials having a higher level of care – the issues of pragmatic trials mentioned in Chapter 4 are particularly pertinent to economic analyses.

Are appropriate inputs and outputs included?

There are several different aspects to the issue of costs. A paper should report which costs have been included and these should be relevant to the question. In simple summary, costs can be:

- direct – the costs associated with the intervention or treatment, acquisition costs, time of professionals involved in care, laboratory costs
- indirect – impact of the ill health on time lost from work or caring activities.

There are a couple of cautions here. First, in health service costings, the term 'direct' cost is used a little differently and excludes overheads (the buildings, the personnel function and so on), whereas, in an economic sense, overheads are part of the direct costs. Second, some authors class all financial impact on the patient as indirect costs (see Earl-Slater and Norwood[14]) whereas, more properly, there are direct and indirect costs for the patient and their family. Drummond *et al.* summarise the direct costs for the patients as out-of-pocket expenses and input into care. The indirect costs are identified as time lost from work and psychological costs – the burden of the disease perhaps.[22]

In costings, two other words are sometimes used – 'tangible' for the easy to measure and 'intangible' for the hard to define.

When examining an economic analysis of a medicine, it can be tempting just to include acquisition costs. This might be acceptable if the options are very similar in delivery and have similar side-effects, but usually a broader approach is required.

Outputs will be measured in a way suitable to the technique. A simple measure is used for CEA, but it should be the important or central measure clinically. For CUA the 'health gain' is examined, for CBA a comprehensive measure of all the consequences or outputs should be included.

In describing costs and benefits, the paper must state which perspective has been used and what has been included. Missing a vital component could change the 'answer'. Thus in a CUA, taking the acquisition costs of a medicine that prevents death used in a critical care context, but ignoring the extended care costs to support the recovery, could understate the cost per QALY considerably.

Discounting

Discounting is the technique used to make adjustments of costs and benefits to allow for the time they occur. In essence, discounting deals with the fact that receiving or spending £1000 today is not the same as knowing you will gain or lose it in 10 years' time. We prefer benefits today and costs tomorrow. Discounting applies an adjusting factor to reflect this. Typically 5% or 6% is applied, so this means in an analysis that a cost of £100 falling today is equal to a cost of £95 or £94 falling in one year's time. Drummond, in *Principles of Economic Appraisal in Healthcare*, gives a fuller description and worked examples of discounting.[24] If all the benefits and costs fall in year 1, discounting is not required.

Although it is generally accepted that future costs should be discounted, discounting future health gains is disputed. Van der Pol and Cairns provide an interesting discussion of the problems of investigating whether people have the same attitude to a health gain as they do to a financial one with respect to timing.[25] For medicines management purposes, the key question is whether applying discounting or adjusting the rate has an important impact on the 'answer'.[26] The analysis should state how these issues have been handled.

Are the issues of the margin addressed?

This is explored in the introductory section of the chapter. It is important that there is clarity in the analyses and how the results are applied. The extra benefits at the extra costs by changing to a new medicine must be considered.

Is a sensitivity analysis performed?

Sensitivity analyses explore how the conclusion of a study alters if some of the variables or assumptions are changed. Thus if treatment A is seen to be more cost-effective than treatment B, given the results of a study, what happens if the study has overestimated the effect of A by 5% or 10%? In a CUA, how would the results look if there were a change in response rate? Good economic analyses will explore these issues. If they do not, the reader or prescribing committee should.

Sensitivity analysis can be undertaken in various ways; the detail will depend on the study design and the factors involved. Briggs, Sculpher and Buxtier provide a useful introduction to sensitivity analysis related to economic evaluations in their 1994 article in *Health Economics*.[26] Table 5.3 provides a brief description of the different types of sensitivity analysis.

Is the analysis appropriate for the local situation?

Generalisability and local application are just as important with economic evaluations as they are with clinical trials regarding effectiveness. In fact, there are more reasons to be wary where costs and benefits are concerned. A medicine seen as having a good cost–benefit profile in a trial setting may not translate into local practice. An example would be a trial where a large part of the benefits of a new medicine derive from hospital admission avoidance but the local situation has already models of care that avoid such episodes. The new treatment could put costs up, not down. Many of the other factors of generalisability of trials also apply to economic evaluations.

Table 5.3 Sensitivity analyses in economic evaluations

Type of sensitivity analysis	Outline description
One way	The results are examined with the adjustment of one variable or assumption, e.g. acquisition cost, response rate
Multi-way	The results are examined with the adjustment of more than one variable or assumption at the same time
Analysis of extremes	The most optimistic and pessimistic results or assumptions are built in to see if the analysis draws the same conclusion. This could be the upper end of a confidence interval or the 'worst' result from a group of trials
Threshold analysis	This explores the question: 'What value does the variable or assumption need to be given for the conclusion to flip?' i.e. If A is more cost-effective than B based on our data, what price would A have to go up to make B more cost-effective? and so on
Probabilistic	This approach plays chance into results, a range of values are explored for each variable or assumption and a probability attached to each of those values. This is a complex technique and methods such as Monte Carlo simulation are used

Monte Carlo simulations run through scenarios repeatedly adjusting variables simultaneously but in patterns according to their predicted probability (for example using an assumed normal distribution curve). The answer produced is a range of results each with a given probability.

Applying health economics

One of the difficulties in using health economics to inform strategic medicines management decisions is the lack of good quality analyses relevant to the question being considered. It is argued that the best form of analysis is one performed alongside an RCT.[27] These will almost certainly not be available early in a medicine's life cycle. To overcome this, economic models are developed; O'Brien called them potential Frankenstein's monsters – taking the parts from many different sources – but that they could be preferred to the vampire-like nature of analyses attached to RCTs, where they suck out the value and distort the work.[28]

An economic model does derive data from various sources and, along with declared assumptions, explores them in terms of inputs and outputs for an intervention. An example would be where to derive a cost per QALY when no economic analyses exist. Data regarding survival are taken from a trial, supported by typical NHS costs for the intervention,

Table 5.4 The Wessex Development and Evaluation Committee's guide for contracting. Cost per life year gained or equivalent

Level of evidence	Below £3000	£3–20,000	Over £20,000	Negative utility
Strong, including RCTs	Strongly recommended	Strongly recommended	Beneficial but high cost	Not recommended
Reasonable	Strongly recommended	Recommended	Beneficial but high cost	Not recommended
Expert opinion	Recommended	Beneficial but high cost	Beneficial but high cost	Not recommended
Inadequate	Not proven	Not proven	Not proven	Not proven

Each entry states the advice to purchasers. Costs were as at 1995.
RCT = randomised controlled trial.

then blended with assumptions or expert opinion on the health-related quality of life. This approach has dangers, but if the sources and assumptions are clearly stated and sensitivity analysis performed, economic models can inform the decision-making process.

Economic models are increasingly popular with pharmaceutical companies, who use them to demonstrate the value of their products. Companies may have in-house health economists or use academic groups. Two important models for interferon beta in multiple sclerosis were the Kendrick and Johnson paper and the 20-year projection model from Swansea and Schering (Phillips *et al.*).[29,30] Both models gave considerably lower estimates than earlier work. NICE had previously not recommended use on the balance of clinical and cost-effectiveness.[31]

Local health communities and the wider healthcare community must have the ability to understand and critique such models. The ability to assess models and analyses associated with trials is as important as other critical appraisal skills. The medicines information network across the UK, so valuable in evaluating clinical effectiveness, could offer this additional area of guidance.

The Williams' paper of 1985 was one of the earlier attempts to use CUA to assist with healthcare decision making.[10] Ten years later members of the Wessex Development and Evaluation Committee wrote up their experience of CUA used to inform contracting of healthcare.[32] ('Contracting' was the term in regular use when the purchaser–provider split was introduced; the term 'commissioning' replaced it.) They noted that such techniques were still in their infancy but attempted to provide 'purchasers' of NHS services with a guide that should receive attention.

Their system included a matrix of four levels of evidence and four levels of cost–utility. Table 5.4 reports this information. They used 'life year gained or equivalent' as their output measure rather than QALY. In essence, where the cost per life year gained exceeded £20,000, the Committee stated the medicine was beneficial but high cost. These were at 1995 costs. Their 'not recommended' category was reserved for treatments that had a 'negative utility' – they did more harm than good would be a crude way to describe this.

In 1997, Cooke, Walley and Drummond reported how far health economics had begun to influence decisions regarding medicines, in hospital practice.[33] Their results of a postal survey of chief pharmacists (2002 replies: 52%) showed fewer than a fifth of respondents had received formal health economics training – much lower than for public health doctors, they noted. They found that the eight pharmaco-economics papers on which they asked questions had had limited influence on advice or actions in hospital. The most influential paper was a cost-effectiveness analysis comparing two ulcer treatments.

Also in 1997, Jantreght *et al.* reported a type of cost–consequences methodology for taking formulary decisions.[34] A number of features of a group of medicines are selected, then each one in the group is rated against each feature. Such systems have merits for choice within a group, but do not address the allocative efficiency or priority-setting questions.

Stephens reported Southampton's attempts to use CUA to inform their investment programme for new medicines.[35] From 1998 to 1989 the hospitals trust in Southampton ranked development bids in terms of cost per QALY, in addition to examining the strength of evidence of effect. They did report CUA data difficult to find and made local estimates to support the process. It was clear CUA was not used as a single deciding factor on any bid.

As described in Chapter 1, the most well-known use of health economic analysis for medicines is in support of NICE evaluations. Technology appraisals summarise the models or studies available to the review panel and state estimates of cost per QALY, among other data. The approach taken is that no single cost-effectiveness threshold exists. It is, however, argued in a King's Fund/Office of Health Economics publication, that their approach implies that technologies achieving a cost of less than £30,000 per QALY will be favourably viewed.[36] The same publication provides an interesting analysis of decisions taken by NICE and the special considerations given to technologies with higher cost per QALY but other particular benefits.

The place of health economics

Chapter 4 explores the hurdles for medicines – efficacy, effectiveness, cost-effectiveness and affordability. A critical review of the evidence of effectiveness enables the local health community to know what the likely health gain will be and how strong the evidence is. The additional step of examining health economic analyses can explore what will be gained from the monies committed in terms of cost–effect, cost–utility or cost–benefit ratio. Ranking priorities on the basis of cost per QALY, or developing a guide to a threshold, is far from perfect and is hampered by a lack of data, but it is a systematised approach to help the process.

An additional application of health economics is programme budgeting with marginal analysis. This is where use of resources is examined and consideration given to switching from one service to another. The purpose of the switching is to increase allocative efficiency by disinvesting in one area providing few benefits from the resources used and investing in another area rich in benefits. In some ways this has been done without an economic label – use of formularies and attempts to reduce 'less worthwhile' medicine use. This approach would not be easy to undertake, especially where reasonably effective medicines were curtailed to invest in others with greater benefit. However, in times of financial pressure it is a technique worth consideration.

Whether or not redistribution of resources among programmes is pursued, local organisations and prescribing committees need access to the appropriate health economic papers. Skills in appraisal and interpretation of those papers are essential. Ideally, there should be capacity to develop simple health economic models. Organisations should consider how to raise the understanding of this subject and develop skills to apply it effectively. Certainly the pharmaceutical industry is aware of this need and invests in modelling to support their marketing efforts.

References

1. Robbins L C. *Essay on the Nature and Significance of Economic Science.* 1932.
2. Samuelson P. *Economics.* Maidenhead: McGraw-Hill, 1976.
3. Allen R, ed. *The Penguin English Dictionary.* London: Penguin, 2001.
4. Donaldson C, Gerard K. *Economics of Healthcare Financing: the Visible Hand.* London: Macmillan, 1993.
5. Department of Health. *The New NHS: Modern, Dependable.* London: The Stationery Office, 1997.
6. Department of Health. *Saving Lives: Our Healthier Nation.* London: The Stationery Office, 1999.

7. Mooney G. *Key Issues in Health Economics.* Hemel Hempstead: Prentice Hall/Harvester Wheatsheaf, 1994.

8. National Prescribing Centre. *An Introduction to Health Economics* MeReC Briefing, Numbers 13 and 14, 2000.

9. Gray A, Vale L. Economic evaluation for decision-making. In Scott A, Maynard A, Elliot R, eds. *Advances in Health Economics.* Chichester: Wiley, 2003.

10. Williams A. Economics of coronary artery bypass grafting. *Br Med J* 1985; 291: 326–329.

11. Kind P, Rosser R, Williams A. Valuation of quality of life: some psychometric evidence. In Jones-Lee M, ed. *The Value of Life and Safety.* Amsterdam: Elsevier, 1982.

12. EuroQol. http://www.euroqol.org (accessed 15 December 2004).

13. Dolin P, Guidex C, Kind P, Williams A. A social tariff for the Euroquol: results from a UK general population survey. *Health Economic Discussion Paper.* York, 1995.

14. Earl-Slater A, Norwood J. Health economic and public health aspects of drug usage. In Panton R, Chapman S, eds. *Medicines Management.* London: BMJ Publishing Group and Pharmaceutical Press, 1998.

15. Brazier J, Deverill M, Green C. A review of the use of health status measures in economic evaluation. *Journal of Health Service Research Policy* 1999; 4: 174–184.

16. National Institute for Clinical Excellence. *Technology Appraisal No. 55: Guidance on the Use of Paclitaxel in the Treatment of Ovarian Cancer.* London: NICE, 2002.

17. Robinson R. Cost–benefit analysis. *Br Med J* 1993; 307: 924–926.

18. Donaldson D. Willingness to pay for publicly provided goods. *Journal of Health Economics* 1990; 9: 103–118.

19. O'Brien B, Gafni A. When do the 'dollars' make sense? *Medical Decision Making* 1996; 16: 288–289.

20. Donaldson C, Shackley P. Willingness to pay for health care. In Scott A, Maynard A, Elliot R, eds. *Advances in Health Economics.* Chichester: Wiley, 2003.

21. Wiffen P. *Evidence-based Pharmacy.* Oxford: Radcliffe Medical Press, 2001.

22. Drummond M, Stoddart G, Torrance G. *Methods for the Economic Evaluation of Health Care Programmes.* Oxford: Oxford University Press, 1987.

23. Haycox A, Walley T. Pharmacoeconomics: evaluating the evaluators. *Br J Clin Pharmacol* 1997; 43: 451–456.

24. Drummond M. *Principles of Economic Appraisal in Health Care.* Oxford: Oxford Medical Publications, 1980.

25. van der Pol M, Cairns J. Methods of eliciting time preferences over future health events. In Scott A, Maynard A, Elliot R, eds. *Advances in Health Economics.* Chichester: Wiley, 2003.

26. Briggs A, Sculpher M, Buxtier M. Uncertainty in the economic evaluation of health care technologies: the role of sensitivity analysis. *Health Econ* 1994; 3: 95–104.

27. Drummond M. *Economic Analysis Alongside Controlled Trials.* London: DH, 1994.

28. O'Brien B. Economic evaluations of pharmaceuticals: Frankenstein's monster or vampire of trials. *Medical Care* 1996; 34 (suppl): DS99–108.

29. Kendrick M, Johnson K. Long term treatment of multiple sclerosis with interferon-β may be cost effective. *Pharmacoeconomics* 2000; 18: 45–53.

30. Phillips C, Gilmour L, Gale R, Palmer M. A cost-utility model of interferon beta-1b in the treatment of relapsing–remitting multiple sclerosis. *J Med Econ* 2001; 4: 35–50.

31. National Institute for Clinical Excellence. *Technology Appraisal No. 32: Beta-Interferon and Glatiramer Acetate for Multiple Sclerosis.* London: NICE, 2002.

32. Stevens A, Colin-Jones D, Gabby J. Quick and clean: authoritative health technology assessment for local health contracting. *Health Trends* 1995; 27: 37–42.

33. Cooke J, Walley T, Drummond M. The use of health economics by hospital pharmacist decision makers – a survey of UK chief pharmacists. *Pharm J* 1997; 259: 779–781.

34. Jantreght R, Van Schlock B, Smith J, de Leeuw P. ACE inhibitors and angiotensin II agents for treatment of hypertension: drugs selected by means of the SOJA method. *Eur Hosp Pharm* 1997; 3: 47–58.

35. Stephens M. Economic analyses to assist drug entry decision making. *Pharm Manage* 2001; 17: 36–40.

36. Towse A, Pritchard C, Devlin N. *Cost-effectiveness Thresholds: Economic and Ethical Issues.* London: King's Fund and Office of Health Economics, 2002.

6

Guidelines

'For a national public service like the NHS there are unacceptable variations in performance and practice' – so declared the Department of Health as the quality initiative encompassing clinical governance was launched.[1] Details of the National Institute for Clinical Excellence (NICE) and the Commission for Health Improvement were also provided. Some of the key concerns identified were:

- lack of clarity on which intervention was most appropriate in a given situation
- research-based changes in practice implemented too slowly
- accepted best practice not always followed.

Chapter 1 discusses the role of NICE with respect to ensuring equity and availability of appraised technologies, but the need for local guidelines was also stated by the Department of Health as a means of delivering consistently good care. However, the document describing these important changes, *A First Class Service*, also mentioned the need to ensure that treatment suited the individual patient: 'Each patient is different and treatment must be tailor-made for their specific needs'. This could be perceived as a paradox – consistent application of evidence for all but individual treatment plans for each. Whether this potential paradox causes a problem depends somewhat on our view of what a guideline is. Balancing the 'usual approach' with individual need is the interface between strategic medicines management and pharmaceutical care. This tension does not apply to guidelines alone; it will crop up in considering new drug entry, formularies and in other aspects of strategic medicines management.

This chapter examines the nature of clinical guidelines. It will briefly explore how their use has developed, consider their production and application and where they can be found. A description of the evidence of their impact and models for their use in medicines management conclude the chapter.

What are guidelines?

Farmer described a guideline as 'a recommendation for patient management that identifies one or more strategies for treatment'.[2] This broad definition suggests that guidelines give advice from those who know, or have examined the evidence, to those faced with decisions regarding patient care; there may be options or only one course of action. In *Clinical Guidelines*, the Department of Health (DH) gave their definition: 'Systematically developed statements which assist clinicians and patients in making decisions about appropriate treatment of specific clinical conditions'.[3] This definition is based on that developed in the United States, recommended by the Agency for Health Care Policy and Research.[4] It is now the definition broadly accepted. In this DH-adopted definition, the idea of recommended strategies is replaced by the thought that the guideline assists decision making – perhaps leaving more to the users of guidelines than is suggested by Farmer's approach. Interestingly, the DH's definition includes the role of the patient in decision making. The various options for treatment in a guideline could be seen as a menu that doctor and patient work through before choosing the intervention to be made.

It would be wrong to make too much of the differences between the definitions mentioned so far, but the apparent differences have been magnified in the debate over guidelines. Wilson summarises the debate as polarised between those who view guidelines as 'a fetter to clinical discretion' leading to medicine by rote, and those who see guidelines as essential in the delivery of good care because of the way they reduce variation in practice.[5] The argument that guidelines are problematic, because of their restriction on clinical freedom, is countered by Tuffnell.[6] He points out that any such document should not be followed unquestioningly, but rather should provide a framework for the thinking clinician. Circumstances may present that require divergence from the usual approach – Tuffnell notes that more experienced staff will be more comfortable in dealing with this, whereas 'junior staff' may not. They would need to seek more experienced advice. This would be typical of practice in secondary care where doctors in training seek support from seniors when needed. An interesting comment is also made, that where divergence takes place, the reasons should be recorded. This hints at issues of liability and responsibility; it suggests clinicians may be asked to justify why decisions were made, at a later stage.

Combining Farmer's and the DH's comments, clinical guidelines can be seen as providing a recommended framework to help professionals and patients decide on the best course of action. How they are derived is another aspect of the definition that differs between Farmer and the DH. The phrase 'systematically developed' is used in *Clinical Guidelines* from the DH.[3] The implication here is that a clear methodology is used in preparing the statement. Perhaps an approach written down by experienced individuals based on their own know-how would fall short of being a clinical guideline, even if it were good advice. An evidence base, which has been examined, is required. The strength of the evidence may vary. Smith suggested a continuum between 'expert guidelines' – where the evidence is the opinion of experienced clinicians – through to 'evidence-based guidelines' – presumably with varying degrees of robustness.[7]

Chapter 4 addresses the way in which evidence can be appraised and the types of evidence sought for medicines management decisions. It is worthwhile revisiting some aspects in the context of guidelines. A descriptive approach has been used to grade the recommendations in guidelines, based on the levels of evidence. The Scottish Intercollegiate Guidelines Network (SIGN) uses grades A–D, based on levels of evidence 1++, through to 4, with eight points in all.[8] Thus a grade A guideline would be one where there is a meta-analysis or systematic review or a randomised controlled trial with a very low risk of bias (1++ level of evidence), such a review/analysis/trial being directly applicable to the population for whom the treatment guideline is designed. This is quite a tough standard, but desirable, if multiple future treatments are to be based on the advice. An alternative way to achieve grade A is given which is equally taxing: allowing 'a body of evidence consisting principally of studies rated as 1+' and being directly applicable. Evidence at 1+ would be of randomised controlled trials with a low, rather than very low, risk of bias. Grades B, C and D are also defined by SIGN, with D being guidelines based on non-analytic studies (level 3 evidence), or on expert opinion.

In a similar way, Tuffnell and Wright use three categories, A–C, and a six-point, evidence-grading scale.[9] This is the same as included in the NICE document issued in 2001, describing their guideline-development process.[10] Guidelines in category A, those that can be used with most confidence, require at least one good randomised control trial relevant to the guideline. Those in category B use randomised controlled trial-derived evidence but not directly applicable. Category C would be a guideline based on expert evidence. Additionally they note 'good practice point' as a fourth aspect of guidance, one that emerges from the guideline group during the development of the guideline.

Guidelines can be seen as tools to assist healthcare professionals and patients in providing diagnoses, treatment and care. They vary in their evidence base. They seek to bring consistency, without stifling individual analysis and thought, particularly where the unexpected or unusual occurs.

Guidelines come in a variety of guises and deal with a number of aspects of healthcare. Thus there are treatment decision focused guidelines – which medicine, what dose? There are those dealing with processes – when should a general practitioner refer a patient to secondary care or when should a pharmacist refer a patient to a general practitioner? There are numerous publications that include guidelines. Smith presents a collection of them in *Guide to Guidelines*, and includes one on asthma, one on back pain and one on cervical cytology.[7] Another example is *Guidelines*, published regularly and providing a collection of guidelines aimed at primary and shared care, many including specific prescribing recommendations.[11] The emphasis of this chapter is guidelines where medicines play a significant part, although the principles of development and use would apply widely.

The place of guidelines in strategic medicines management

Guidelines are an important feature of strategic medicines management. *A Spoonful of Sugar* includes guidelines as an important part of a drugs and therapeutic committee's function and, as discussed in Chapter 3, implies that formularies should include guidance on medicine use.[12] Their purpose is to provide a summary of the evidence in a way that supports good practice. They could strengthen the formulary by adding value to the document and by setting out the various agents' roles in therapy. They aim to educate and to provide a framework to help decision in the majority of cases. This means that they can support individual treatment without dictating individual decisions – in the way that Figure I.2 identified how strategic medicines management supports pharmaceutical care. How well these aims are achieved will be addressed later in a brief review of the evidence on guidelines.

How did guidelines emerge?

Farmer traced the emergence of guidelines to the USA of the 1960s.[2] The motivation was seen as a desire to control costs, standardising treatment to avoid unexpected expenditure. However, Farmer also gives other reasons for their development, both in the USA and in the United Kingdom. The need to reduce risk and to improve quality by reducing variation is probably an equally important driver. This can also influence cost. Farmer also mentions the desire for educational tools and regulation as reasons for development.

Littlejohns points to the expansion of clinical audit in the late 1980s as a key impetus for guidelines in the UK.[13] Audit requires defined standards; guidelines can provide these. Various bodies were, and remain, involved with guideline development, including the Royal Colleges. One set of guidelines where prescribing decisions are central and which has a considerable history are the asthma guidelines, published in the *British Medical Journal* in 1990.[14,15] This was the combined work of the British Thoracic Society, the Royal College of Physicians of London, the King's Fund Centre and the National Asthma Campaign. In 2003 the British Thoracic Society, jointly with SIGN, with partner organisations, published the *British Guideline on the Management of Asthma,* familiar to users of the *British National Formulary.*[16,17]

Other guidelines were developed during the 1990s, often with medical college engagement. An example is when, in July 1995, the NHS Executive commissioned the Royal College of General Practitioners' Quality Improvement Group to develop evidence based guidelines for primary care on the management of low back pain. This was aimed at the range of clinicians involved in first-contact care.[18]

The NHS Executive further promoted guidelines with its 1996 document, *Clinical Guidelines*, as mentioned earlier.[3] Then *A First Class Service* restated their role in improving the consistency of care.[1] Subsequently, as described in Chapter 1, NICE has reviewed and endorsed a number of guidelines and continues to support their use as means of standard setting in healthcare. Some are inherited or adapted, and others have been specifically developed by NICE.[19]

How are guidelines developed and used?

The nature and content of the guideline

The *Dictionary of Evidence-based Medicine* identifies nine information sets that guidelines ought to include, derived from work in America.[4,20] The list includes stating the purpose of the guideline, what evidence has been used and how the outcomes sought were valued. More mundane, but essential, items are also mentioned such as the date reviews were undertaken. Box 6.1 provides the full list. In summary, the guideline should make it clear what advice, for which circumstances, is being given by whom, how that advice has been derived and from what evidence. The asthma guidelines mentioned earlier can be examined using the checklist and be seen to have each of these features, to some degree at least.[16] Table 6.1 gives some examples of how this is achieved.

Box 6.1 Information that should be included in guidelines.

- Purpose of guideline and reasons for developing
- Options that were considered
- The clinical and economic outcomes that were sought by applying the guideline
- What evidence was there and how it was collected and synthesised
- Who valued the outcomes and how
- The benefits, disbenefits and costs
- How the guideline has been reviewed and validated
- Any relevant sponsor or interest
- Date last revised

In addition to the guideline content, thought has been given to the characteristics of a good guideline. *Effective Health Care*[21] identified eleven attributes of good guidelines and these were restated in the NHS Executive's *Clinical Guidelines*.[3] There is some correlation between the attributes list and the content list mentioned earlier. For example, both point to the requirement for review date and process. Good guidelines are seen as those where correctly interpreted, relevant and recent evidence is used. Two questions are asked: 'Would another group derive the same guidance given the same evidence?' And second: 'Would different professionals interpret and use the guideline in the same way?' These are not easily answered without experiment. If ambiguity, in the evidence or in the guideline wording, can be identified, the answer could be *no*. Any guideline writer would be well-advised to reflect on these questions during the development process before dissemination. Clarity of language is given as another desirable attribute. Perhaps more interestingly a further attribute is that the guideline should tend to lead to improvements in health at acceptable costs, the 'acceptable costs' bringing in a health economic perspective – will the guideline improve 'bang for buck' or, more accurately, will it 'bring a bigger bang at a price worth paying?'

The nature and key features of guidelines have been discussed in the literature and examples of good guidelines can be found. *Bandolier* points readers to a good anticoagulant guideline but also points to the variability of guidelines that get produced.[22,23] The article highlights several reviews of guidelines, including Thomson *et al.* who published their findings on the variability of anticoagulant guidelines in 1998.[24] The study comprised a postal survey regarding anticoagulant guidelines

Table 6.1 Checklist for the British guideline on the management of asthma[15]

Feature	How the guideline achieves
Purpose of guideline and reasons for developing	The introduction states the history of the guideline and its aim
Options that were considered	Treatment choices are stated with the levels of evidence found, e.g. section 5.5 deals with how inhaler devices may be chosen
The clinical and economic guidelines that were sought	Various outcomes are identified, e.g. section 12.1.3 The target of normal lung function is given as a good proxy for quality of life
How the evidence was collected and synthesised and what it comprised	The introduction summarises the methodology and refers to the SIGN approach
Who valued the outcomes and how	Who was involved and the evidence used for outcomes are given but no economic evaluation of outcomes is made
The benefits, disbenefits and costs	Safety data are included, e.g. section 4.2.2 discusses the impact of inhaled steroids on children. Outcome data are included which describe successful management. Cost-effectiveness and costs are rarely discussed
How the guideline has been reviewed and validated	Review process is described in the introduction
Any relevant sponsor or interest	The groups involved in supporting the process are given. Interests declared by those involved can be obtained from the SIGN executive
The date last revised	Explained in the introduction

for atrial fibrillation, semi-structured interviews of guideline leads and a practical application of the guidelines found on a group of patients' blood samples. They found 20 guidelines and undertook 15 interviews. In 6 of the 15, groups had been used to develop the guideline; the remainder were single-handed efforts, often with no external review. Only one was described as evidence based. Other features described earlier as indicators of good guidelines were missing. Disturbingly, when the guidelines were applied, extremely varied actions emerged as recommendations. Between 13% and 100% of the patients would have had anticoagulation commenced, depending on which guideline was followed. Thomson concluded: 'The variation in the guidelines is likely to be caused by their non-systematic development'. This supports the argument that to achieve good guidelines, a sound development methodology must be chosen.

Developing a guideline

Tuffnell and Wright state two axioms regarding guidelines – to para-phrase: the better the development plan, the greater the credibility of the guideline; and the greater the users' ownership of the development process, the better the chance it will be put into practice.[9] These prin-ciples are echoed by other writers on the subject of guidelines, who also emphasise the need for a systematic approach. Hardy points out that local guidelines are likely to gain local acceptance and so be well-used.[25]

A number of development methodologies have been described and used at national and local levels.[9,19,25-27] Although the approach taken by NICE may differ from that in a single organisation in terms of stakeholders, resources available and dissemination, the key features of well-planned guideline development are the same. These have been synthesised in Figure 6.1.

The first step in the development process is idea generation. SIGN cite variation in practice as a key reason to develop a guideline; Tuffnell and Wright suggest findings from the confidential enquiries in perioper-ative death as an important driver for guidelines.[9,28] A further sugges-tion for idea generation is the clinical negligence scheme for trusts. This could be broadened to encompass other risk programmes, particularly at a local level. Organisations do need to learn from complaints, adverse events and compensation claims. One way of improving matters is to develop a pertinent guideline – and ensure that it is used. Pharmacists may have a particularly important role to play in idea generation for prescribing guidelines or guidelines where medicine use is part of a larger subject. In hospital, clinical pharmacist interventions may be a rich source of issues that need action. If junior doctors continually mispre-scribe a particular medicine for a particular condition, a guideline may help educate and improve matters. Shekelle *et al.* add the regular morbidity and mortality meetings to the list of sources for idea gener-ation.[26] They also mention cost as a driver – where practice varies and has big resource implications because of that variation, a guideline may help to improve resource use by reducing variation.

The same subjects that help derive ideas can help prioritise. Resources will be consumed in guideline preparation, more so if done well. Guidelines that provide biggest benefits should be addressed first. SIGN state that their guideline subjects are chosen only if the following three conditions apply: there is a strong research base, there is a vari-ation in practice that has an impact on outcome, and the production of a guideline is expected to improve matters.[27]

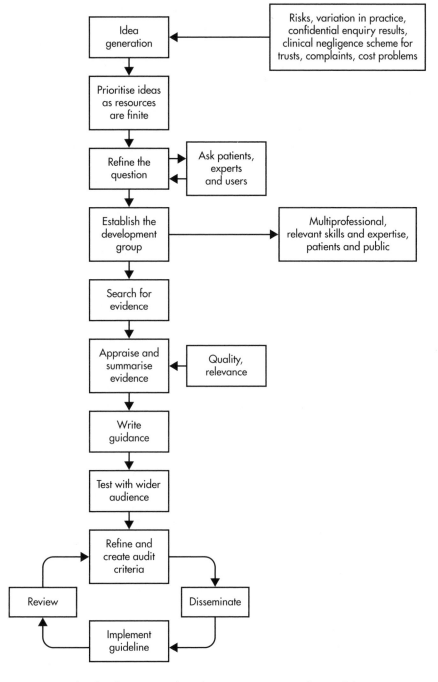

Figure 6.1 The development and implementation process for guidelines.

The third step towards guideline production is to refine the 'question' being addressed. This process can benefit from involvement of patients, experts and potential users. Certainly, key stakeholders' involvement (particularly for local guidelines) at this stage, is likely to help develop ownership among the target audience. Presumably for national or 'multicommunity' guidelines, the involvement of 'members of each tribe' in development will help later at the application stage, that is, where physicians or clinical pharmacists or midwives are part of the development group, their peers will feel more comfortable in adopting the guidelines.

Once the question is clear, development can begin. A mixture of the range of stakeholders and the range of skills is needed when a group is formed. The number involved must be manageable (Shekelle *et al.* suggest between 6 and 15) and will vary with the complexity of the guideline and the intended range of users.[26] Patient involvement is desirable, particularly if we think of the definition of a guideline: 'Helping professionals and patients decide a course of action'. Tuffnell and Wright suggest health service managers as members as they will be overseeing the implementation of guidelines and may need to support resource allocation to allow that implementation.[9] However, this may be a poor use of time, so long as the guideline group keep in mind issues such as affordability.

The skills required for a development group include literature searching, critical appraisal, statistical, health service research and health economics. An understanding of how to organise a project and of group dynamics as well as writing, editorial and communication skills are all essential but perhaps easily overlooked.

The next stage in the process will be to find the evidence. The process is similar to that described in Chapter 4 regarding managed entry of medicines. Shekelle *et al.* suggest a hierarchy to follow when preparing guidelines:

- Seek systematic reviews relevant to the question.
- Check for current Cochrane review groups.
- Use MEDLINE, EMBASE and the Cochrane Controlled Trials Register to seek primary sources.[26]

Clearly, if few randomised controlled trials exist, the evidence that is available will need to be searched for.

Critically appraising, summarising and synthesising the evidence must then be undertaken. Key factors in the process are to check the quality and relevance of the data found. The skills identified earlier will be essential in this process. Inevitably, some evidence will conflict with the main body; this needs to be dealt with wisely. NICE emphasise the need for a robust method to bring together the expert views of the evidence.[19] Tuffnell and Wright stress the need for brutal editing if clarity is to be achieved.[9] A worthy but wordy document is less likely to be used than a clear, concise guideline.

An indication of the confidence placed in the recommended options, based on the level of evidence used, will need to be agreed by the group. The NICE and SIGN grades were described earlier in the chapter.

Once ready for the wider world, the guideline should be reviewed and refined. SIGN methodology includes an open meeting followed by independent review.[27] Local guidelines will benefit by comment from medical and other relevant staff, in addition to those on the development group. If not already involved, clinical pharmacologist and microbiologist (where relevant) advice will add to the credibility of the guidelines. Again, if not involved, representatives of the local drug and therapeutic committees or formulary team should be consulted. Issuing a guideline to general practice with medicines not locally approved for use, or to hospital teams for non-formulary items will be counterproductive.

After refinement the document is ready for use. NICE guidelines include key audit criteria; these can be added prior to issue for local guidelines.

Developing a guideline from an idea to a useful document is a major endeavour but those involved will have opportunities to refresh their knowledge or learn new skills. Working in a team to produce the guideline can in itself be a developmental exercise. However, the task is not over at publication. Dissemination and implementation must be done well if the effort of production is not to be wasted.

Dissemination

National guidelines prepared by NICE or SIGN are disseminated using a clear methodology and are accessible via websites. Chapter 1 discusses how local organisations can work with these to improve their strategic medicines management. Wright and Tuffnell suggest that educational meetings involving local opinion leaders can be an excellent method of getting guidelines known.[28] Hudgings described the USA's Agency for Health Care Policy and Research methods of dissemination at a 1995 conference.[29] She identified a distribution process via a clearing house, a quick reference guide published in key journals, use of consumer publications, multimedia products, conference presentations and press releases. Clearly, such an extensive, multifaceted launch would not be appropriate for a local guideline, but the principles of being creative, ensuring that patients and professionals are informed, and that use meetings plus bulletins would apply. Use of the press locally requires careful thought and expert public relations advice but it could be helpful.

For the prescriber, access to the guideline at the point of prescribing is more likely to help adherence than a once-a-year reminder. Here, computerised prescribing support can be of great value, but pocket-book summaries of local guidelines could be just as easy to access.

Tailoring the dissemination to the guideline and to the users is likely to be better than 'one approach suits all'.

Implementation

To a degree, development and dissemination are the first stages of implementation. Development including stakeholders informs and builds support. Dissemination makes access possible. However, ensuring that the guideline is translated into practice is more than simply making it available. For national guidelines there may be important incentives or pressures to use; SIGN describe the 'twin levers' of clinical governance and the Clinical Standards Board for Scotland. For local guidelines there may be levers and incentives, but perhaps not of the same magnitude.

Littlejohns and Humphris describe how implementation of guidelines was undertaken for the South Thames Assisting Clinical Effectiveness Programme.[30] Taking time to plan well, involving clinicians, building the guidelines into education meetings and into organisation-wide audits were seen as the key factors for success.

Bringing in a new guideline is a change management process and, as such, requires effective leadership. As with any change management process, success is more likely if those who need to change see the benefits of that change.

Lombarts adapts professional marketing processes to consider how guidelines can be brought into practice.[31] She describes work in Holland where the 'client sub groups' were approached according to type. Thus, early adopters require just to be informed about the guidelines and what the benefits are. The next group, the majority, will take up the guideline when motivated to do so – seeing peers using it, discussions at meetings. The late adopters will require the incentives or sanctions to implement, as will the 'laggards'. Figure 6.2 puts this into pictorial form.

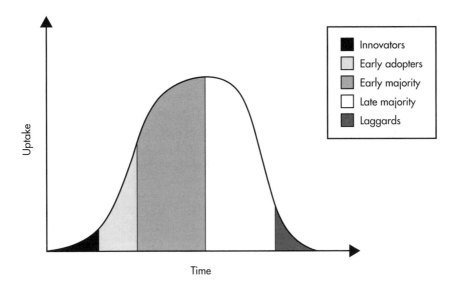

Figure 6.2 The uptake of innovation.

The pharmacist can play an important role in implementation of guidelines that include medicines. Ensuring that doctors or practice staff are aware of the guidelines, making them accessible to prescribers, and intervening if they are not being used, can occur in secondary and primary care. This is particularly true in supporting junior doctors in secondary/tertiary care. Clinical audit can allow a review of adherence and, if run well, audit meetings can provide feedback to improve practice – or allow guideline changes if they are needed.

Do guidelines work?

This chapter places guidelines at the heart of strategic medicines management. The process to develop a good guideline has been described. But do guidelines have the impact sought? What evidence is there? Before addressing the question directly, it is helpful to consider what is meant by a guideline 'working'. Adherence to a guideline may be seen as a prerequisite to it working. This is reasonable, although as discussed earlier, some divergence would be expected. A guideline could have a positive educational role or even change behaviour without achieving adherence. However, to argue the need to create a set of guidelines on this basis does seem rather flimsy.

Another angle on the impact of guidelines would be whether

patients and professionals value them. Returning to the definition –
helping patients and professionals decide – a guideline that was working
might be one that patients felt empowered them in the management of
their disease or care. Further areas of guidelines working relate to their
intended purposes:

- Is safety increased or are adverse events decreased?
- Is practice made more equitable or is consistency increased?
- Are costs controlled or cost-effectiveness increased?
- Do guidelines increase the knowledge or skills of users?

There are many publications assessing the impact of specific guidelines,
adherence to guidelines and ways of changing practice (guidelines being
one such tool). Here, a few examples that relate to the various aspects
described are included.

Coleman and Nicholl undertook a postal survey to gauge the
general attitude to guidelines of medically qualified staff. Directors of
public health, consultants and general practitioners were included.[32] The
mean number of guidelines used by health authority staff was 4.3,
whereas consultants and GPs reported fewer – means of 1.9 and 1.8,
respectively. In the same way, 87% of health authority responders said
their practice had been influenced, whereas 52% of hospital consultants
and 57% of GPs said the same. The report was published in 2001. It
suggests that, although guidelines are in place, 'front-line' staff tended
to use them less than those involved in commissioning. But what
evidence is there of adherence?

A systematic review of evaluations of guidelines, from 1993,
concluded that adherence to guidelines is influenced by their source,
method of dissemination and how users are reminded.[33] Guidelines that
were created locally, were supported by targeted education and were
included in patient-specific 'point of use' reminders, were the most likely
to be successful. National guidelines, issued by publication in journals
with general reminders, were least likely to gain adherence. The review
was, of course, in the pre-NICE era.

Davis and Taylor-Vaisey published a systematic review of underpinning theory and evidence of uptake of guidelines.[34] They found some
evidence of guidelines having an impact on care, but the impact was
small. It was found to depend on six key factors – most of the factors
have been described in discussing good guidelines. Simple guidelines that
are expected to have a big benefit over typical pre-guideline practice
were reported as more likely to achieve adherence. They reported some
evidence that younger clinicians were more responsive to guidelines.

They also found that incentives, regulation and patient pressure assisted adherence.

Turning to a specific area of practice, Bauer reported a review of adherence to mental health guidelines, from literature published in 2000.[35] Nine studies were controlled trials; six of these achieved 'adequate adherence'. Bauer noted that several studies showed that when the 'implementation support' ceased, adherence fell.

Three single studies, rather than reviews, dealing with specific practice areas suggest that adherence tends to be limited. MacClean *et al.* reported at the British Pharmaceutical Conference in 1999 that although GPs claimed to use a Greater Glasgow Health Board guideline on use of statins in hypercholesterolaemia (80% of those surveyed), adherence was poor.[36] Wrong choice of initial dose and inadequate dose titration were reported. More recently Baker *et al.* reported on the application of angina and asthma guidelines – comparing guidelines supported by summaries with guidelines supported by summaries and feedback.[37] They concluded a few interventions were adhered to, but nothing much changed overall – a rather gloomy summary. Bloom *et al.* reported work from the USA, based on monitoring during the period 1995 to 2001, examining compliance to cancer network guidelines on chemotherapy.[38] They found about only 37% of eligible patients received chemotherapy in line with the guideline, further evidence of non-adherence to guidelines.

The evidence suggests that adherence is not easily achieved, even if well-designed, but especially if not well-implemented. Those contemplating guideline introduction need to be confident that the process they intend to follow is going to give the best chance of adherence and that they are making a good use of the resources they intend to expend. There is further evidence of the value and impact of guidelines, which may give the reader more encouragement.

Woolf *et al.* argued that guidelines are seen to have value in terms of empowering patients and in improving consistency in care.[39] National guidelines have a particular role in the latter; Chapter 1 discusses the impact of NICE guidelines. Other studies have shown that doctors value guidelines, for example, the antibiotic guidelines, where they were seen to inform and improve practice.[40] A review of surveys of doctors' attitudes to clinical practice guidelines concluded that consistently high satisfaction levels towards guidelines are reported.[41] The reason given was that clinicians thought guidelines would improve quality. However, concerns were also regularly reported on the practicality of guidelines and the role guidelines have in cutting costs. Perhaps these may be based on the suspicion that the motives for guidelines are not in the patients' best interests.

Moving from the perceived value to the impact on outcomes, another review, published in 1997, looked at the impact of guidelines of patient outcomes in primary care.[42] It was found that 38% of the studies examined demonstrated significant improvements in outcomes, improvements that had resulted from use of the guideline under study. However, improvements tended to be limited, were seen in only some patient groups and did not persist with time. Randomised and non-randomised studies were included. A study published since that review by Wright *et al.* examined the impact of asthma and of angina guidelines in two health authorities in England.[43] A non-random, controlled design was followed. Although the active group had an increased reported awareness of the guidelines, both active and control groups had similar improvements in asthma and angina care. The study concluded that the guideline gave little measurable effect on prescribing behaviour or on hospital admissions. The authors did suggest that patient-specific feedback and ongoing audit to support the guidelines, neither of which were used in the study, might have given improved results.

Binyon and Cooke looked at the literature relating to the impact of antibiotic guidelines on antibiotic resistance.[44] This was not a systematic review, but included examples from around the world of some impact on resistance by introducing antibiotic policies. Guidelines may often be seen as a means of controlling expenditure. Certainly in the context of strategic medicines management this is so, although clearly their role in delivering consistent care and reducing risk is also pertinent.

An early example of a guideline having an effect on use of resources is the *British Medical Journal* report of the impact of guidelines on the use of radiography in hospital.[45] A multicentre trial looked at how Royal College guidelines influenced requests for radiological examinations. They successfully reduced the referral rate, hence exposure and resource use. There are examples of studies examining medicine-related guidelines, but the evidence of reduction in expenditure tends to be limited and the study design not ideal. The McCaig *et al.* and the Binyon papers already mentioned provide some support for the argument that guidelines can help control prescribing costs.[40,44]

Two further papers are worth mention.[46,47] Both concluded that there was little impact on practice of the primary care guidelines examined and that there are significant barriers to use of decision-support systems. Making time during consultation for use of such systems was suggested as a significant obstacle.

Overall then, there is some evidence that guidelines, if designed and implemented well, will have some impact. However, they cannot be seen as a panacea to effective medicines use. It may be that guidelines dealing with prescribing matters are key in strategic medicines management, but getting individual care right requires more than a guideline. This is where the clinical pharmacist and pharmaceutical care can contribute.

Legal aspects of guidelines

It is not within the scope of this book to explore and explain in full the legal issues relating to guidelines, but some mention is essential. A key question that may arise is: 'If things go wrong, does the fact that a guideline was followed or was not followed have an impact?' And for the creators of a guideline: 'What is our liability for things going wrong if the guideline was followed or misinterpreted?'

Tingle argues that guidelines should work to reduce the level of clinical negligence claims by reducing adverse events.[48] He also argues that, in an English tort law context, it would be unlikely that mere divergence from a guideline would itself be viewed as negligence. Of course there may be circumstances where following a guideline, irrespective of circumstances, would itself be negligent. Tingle does give examples of legal cases where national clinical guidelines have been used to support a claim for damages and where a clinician having no knowledge of a widely disseminated guideline is seen as unacceptable. Samanta *et al.* point out that recent cases have illustrated that courts take national guidelines as responsible and reasonable medical practice – implying if they are not followed there ought to be a good reason, preferably recorded in the notes, one assumes.[49]

The NHS Executive's *Clinical Guidelines* included advice for guideline developers to enable them to reduce the risk of legal action arising from their work.[3] This advice includes some of the features described in good guideline development earlier: review dates, multidisciplinary development, clear statement of purpose, written so they are permissive of divergence. Case law is likely to develop on these matters and the issues are not simple. The impact of Bolam, of Bolitho and more recent cases needs to be considered in this context.[50,51] For those leading the local development and use of guidelines, advice on the legal issues or an understanding of their implications would be a useful acquisition.

The local approach to guidelines

The chapter looks at the definition of clinical guidelines, briefly describes their emergence in the UK, examines how they can be developed and disseminated, and looks at some of the evidence of their impact. What should local organisations and health communities do about guidelines? There is a range of responses. One approach would be simply to seek to implement nationally produced guidelines, NICE or SIGN documents, perhaps those from Royal Colleges. Certainly this alone is a significant undertaking. The methodologies are well-described and, generally, there is a solid evidence base. The issue of local ownership could be problematic, but the levers on performance may compensate for this. Even if this is the approach, there will be a need for local application of guidelines. A decision to limit the range of products normally available would mean that some local guidance to supplement NICE documentation is needed. In any case, there will be a need to ensure that nationally produced guidelines are available and implemented; an audit programme should form part of this process. Simple measures, such as how much is spent on statins or on atypical antipsychotic medicines, will be relatively easy to establish. Demonstrating that prescribing is in line with guidelines for all eligible patients is more difficult. Practice, directorate and organisational clinical audit programmes need to pick up these issues, prioritising areas of particular local concern.

Organisations, directorates and practices may feel there are local matters not dealt with in the national guidelines. These, and the tailoring or application of national guidelines, will require local processes to ensure that the standards described earlier in the chapter are met. The aim should be to avoid duplication of effort, while ensuring local relevance and commitment. For guidelines that have relevance almost exclusively in secondary/tertiary care, a hospital's drug and therapeutic committee might be the appropriate ratifying body. Examples could be intravenous potassium replacement for severe hypokalaemia, surgical antibiotic prophylaxis, treating diabetic ketoacidosis and anti-emesis for inpatient chemotherapy treatment. Larger hospitals, with many specialities, may find there are conflicting ideas on what the guidelines should contain or perhaps just have different approaches, which have a reasonable evidence base. In such situations, it may be acceptable to have several guidelines but there are significant risks of confusion and hence errors. Drug and therapeutic committees can act as arbiters and ensure consistency.

Guidelines for use across secondary and primary care require input from both sectors. This helps with ownership and hence with adherence. It also means that a specialist view and a generalist view can be taken into account; the hope of such a fusion is that an evidence-based but pragmatic document can be developed. In England, primary care trusts form a suitably sized health community to work in partnership with a district general hospital, although natural groupings of several primary care trusts may come together to develop guidelines. Individual practice guidelines, informed by secondary care opinion, may also have a role. However, this could mean considerable use of resources and duplication of effort. A compromise could be that a broad guideline, or range of options, gain health community support, with adaptation to practice preference permitted. Primary care governance or prescribing groups could oversee the implementation of guidelines but a joint primary/secondary prescribing committee would be the ideal group to ratify locally adapted or developed guidelines that deal with medicines.

Medicines information pharmacists, particularly those with critical appraisal skills, have an important part to play in examining and summarising the evidence to prepare guidelines. Medical staff from secondary and primary care, not just those working closely in the relevant field, are also essential players. As discussed earlier in the chapter and in Chapter 2 regarding committees, patient or public involvement is important, although at the time of writing, still a group that organisations find hard to engage systematically.

Once put in place, there need to be systems to ensure that latest copies are available, regular reviews occur and a definitive index is available. Using web technology would seem to be the answer, even if desktop or junior doctor pocket versions of guidelines are more easily accessed in less IT-rich organisations.

Guidelines that help prescribers and patients make good choices about therapy, that assist in controlling costs and that improve standards have an important role in strategic medicines management. They take considerable resources to produce, although there are increasing numbers of high-quality national guidelines available, which may need little or no local tailoring. Writing them may be difficult but getting them to work is harder. There is evidence of their success, but there is also evidence of them making moderate or negligible impact. Choosing the right area to target, good planning and persistent application should be foremost in the minds of those seeking to ensure that effective guidelines help organisations make the most of their medicines.

References

1. Department of Health. *A First Class Service: Quality in the New NHS.* London: DH, 1998.
2. Farmer A. Medical practice guidelines: lessons from the United States. *Br Med J* 1993; 307: 313–317.
3. NHS Executive. *Clinical Guidelines: Using Clinical Guidelines to Improve Patient Care within the NHS.* London: DH, 1996.
4. Field M, Kohr K, eds. *Guidelines for Clinical Practice. From Development to Use.* Washington DC: National Academy Press, 1992.
5. Wilson J. In Tingle J, Foster C, eds. *Clinical Guidelines: Law, Policy and Practice.* London: Cavendish, 2002: 1.
6. Tuffnell D. In Tingle J, Foster C, eds. *Clinical Guidelines: Law, Policy and Practice.* London: Cavendish, 2002: 24.
7. Smith P, ed. *Guide to the Guidelines: Disease Management Made Simple*, 2nd edn. Abingdon: Radcliffe Medical Press, 1996.
8. Scottish Intercollegiate Guidelines Network. Methodology for evidence review. http://www.sign.ac.uk/methodology/agreeguide/agree/grading_system.html (accessed 8 December 2004).
9. Tuffnell D, Wright J. In Tingle J, Foster C, eds. *Clinical Guidelines: Law, Policy and Practice.* London: Cavendish, 2002: 44–46.
10. National Institute for Clinical Excellence. *The Guideline Development Process – Information for National Collaborating Centres and Guideline Development Groups, No. 040.* London: Oaktree Press, 2001.
11. Foord-Kelcey G, ed. *Guidelines Volume 21.* Berkhampstead: Medendium Group, 2003.
12. Audit Commission. *A Spoonful of Sugar: Medicines Management in NHS Hospitals.* London: Audit Commission, 2001.
13. Littlejohns P. In Humphris D, Littlejohns P, eds. *Implementing Clinical Guidelines: a Practical Guide.* Abingdon: Radcliffe Medical Press, 1999: 3–4.
14. Thoracic Society, Research Unit (Royal College of Physicians of London), King's Fund Centre, National Asthma Campaign. Guidelines for management of asthma in adults: 1 – chronic persistent asthma. *Br Med J* 1990; 301: 651–653.
15. Thoracic Society, Research Unit (Royal College of Physicians of London), King's Fund Centre, National Asthma Campaign. Guidelines for management of asthma in adults: 2 – acute severe asthma. *Br Med J* 1990; 301: 797–800.
16. British Thoracic Society, Scottish Intercollegiate Guidelines Network. British guideline on the management of asthma: a national clinical guideline. *Thorax* 2003; 58 (suppl 1).
17. British Medical Association and the Royal Pharmaceutical Society. *British National Formulary*, 47th edn, London: BMA and RPS, 2004.
18. Royal College of General Practice. Backpain guidelines. http://www.rcgp.org.uk/clinspec/guidelines/backpain/backpain5.asp (now unavailable).
19. NICE website. http://www.nice.org.uk/catcg2.asp?c=20034 (accessed 8 December 2004)
20. Li Wan Po A. *The Dictionary of Evidenced-Based Medicine.* Abingdon: Radcliffe Medical Press, 1998.

21. Anon. Implementing clinical practice guidelines. *Effective Health Care Bulletin No. 8*. Leeds: University of Leeds, 1994.

22. *Bandolier*, 102-2. Anticoagulant guideline. http://www.jr2.ox.ac.uk/bandolier/band102/b102-2.html (accessed 8 December 2004).

23. *Bandolier*. Variability of guidelines. http://www.jr2.ox.ac.uk/bandolier/booth/AF/flow.html (accessed 8 December 2004).

24. Thomson R, McElray H, Sudlow M. Guidelines on anticoagulant treatment for artrial fibrillation in Great Britain: variation in content and implications for treatment. *Br Med J* 1998; 316: 509–513.

25. Hardy N. Developing and implementing clinical guidelines in primary care. *Pharm J* 1996; 256: 757–759.

26. Shekelle P, Woolf S, Eccles M, Grimshaw J. Developing clinical guidelines. *Br Med J* 1999; 318: 593–596.

27. Scottish Intercollegiate Guidelines Network. Methodology for guideline development. http://www.sign.ac.uk/about/introduction.html (accessed 8 December 2004).

28. Wright J, Tuffnell D. In Tingle J, Foster C, eds. *Clinical Guidelines: Law, Policy and Practice*. London: Cavendish, 2002: 53–73.

29. Hudgings C. Guideline development and dissemination programme: Agency for Health Care Policy and Research, USA. In Deighan M, Hitch S. *Clinical Effectiveness from Guidelines to Cost Effective Practice*. Brentwood: Earlybrave Publications, 1995: 65–70.

30. Littlejohns P, Humphris D. How effective are clinical guidelines? In Humphris D, Littlejohns P, eds. *Implementing Clinical Guidelines: a Practical Guide*. Abingdon: Radcliffe Medical Press, 1999: 7–12.

31. Lombarts K. Dutch physicians using external peer review in implementing and evaluating clinical guidelines. In Deighan M, Hitch S. *Clinical Effectiveness from Guidelines to Cost Effective Practice*. Brentwood: Earlybrave Publications, 1995: 59–63.

32. Coleman P, Nicholl J. Influence of evidence based guidance on health policy and clinical practice in England. *Qual Health Care* 2001; 10: 229–237.

33. Grimshaw J, Russell I. Effect of clinical guidelines on medical practice: a systematic review of rigorous evaluations. *Lancet* 1993; 342: 1317–1322.

34. Davis D, Taylor-Vaisey A. Translating guidelines into practice. A systematic review of theoretic concepts, practical experience and research evidence in the adoption of clinical, practice guidelines. *Can Med Assoc J* 1997; 157: 408–416.

35. Bauer M. A review of quantitative studies of adherence to mental health guidelines. *Harvard Rev Psychiatr* 2002; 10: 138–153.

36. McLean F, Bayter A, Lee A, Morrison C. Statin prescribing in primary care and GP's perception of hypercholesterolaemia. *Pharm J* 1999: R 4–5.

37. Baker R, Fraser R, Store M *et al.* Randomised controlled trial of the impact of guidelines, prioritised review criteria and feedback on implementation of recommendations for angina and asthma. *Br J Gen Pract* 2003; 53: 284–291.

38. Bloom B, de Pouvourille N, Chhatre S *et al.* Breast cancer treatment in clinical practice compared to best evidence and practice guidelines. *Br J Cancer* 2004; 90: 26–30.

39. Woolf S, Gray R, Hutchinson A. *et al.* Potential benefits, limitations and harms of clinical guidelines. *Br Med J* 1999; 318: 527–530.

40. McCaig D, Hind C, Downie G, Wilkinson S. Antibiotic use in elderly hospital inpatients before and after the introduction of treatment guidelines. *Int J Pharm Pract* 1999; 7: 18–28.

41. Farquhar C, Kofa E, Slutsky J. Clinicians' attitudes to clinical practice guidelines: a systematic review. *Med J Aust* 2002; 177: 502–506.

42. Worrall G, Chaulk P, Freake D. The effects of clinical practice guidelines on patient outcomes in primary care: a systematic review. *Can Med Assoc J* 1997; 156: 1705–1712.

43. Wright J, Warren E, Reeves J. *et al*. Effectiveness of multifaceted implementation of guidelines in primary care. *J Health Serv Res Policy* 2003; 8: 142–148.

44. Binyon D, Cooke R. Restrictive antibiotic policies – how effective are they? *Hosp Pharm* 2000; 7: 183–187.

45. Royal College of Radiologists Working Party. Influence of Royal College of Radiologists' guidelines on hospital practice: a multicentre trial. *Br Med J* 1992; 304: 740–743.

46. Eccles M, McCall E, Steen N *et al*. Effect of computerised evidence based guidelines on management of asthma and angina in adults in primary care: cluster randomised controlled trial. *Br Med J* 2002: 325: 941–947.

47. Rosseau N, McColl E, Newton J *et al*. Practice based, longitudinal, qualitative interview study of computerised evidence based guidelines in primary care. *Br Med J* 2003; 326: 314–321.

48. Tingle J. The developing role of clinical guidelines. In Tingle J, Foster C, eds. *Clinical Guidelines: Law, Policy and Practice*. London: Cavendish, 2002: 99–110.

49. Samanta A, Samanta J, Gunn M. Legal consideration of clinical guidelines: will NICE make a difference? *J R Soc Med* 2003; 96: 133–138.

50. *Bolam v. Friern Hospital Management Committee* [1957] 2 All ER 118, 112.

51. *Bolitho v. City and Hackney Health Authority* (1993) 13 BMLR 111.

7

Systematic approaches to strategic medicines management

The use of medicines in a health community is a complex activity. There are many thousands of prescribing and 'administering or taking' events each day. Choices are made with respect to dose, route, form, product, chemical entity, timing and so on. There are hundreds of prescribers, purchasers and thousands of recipients of medicines. There are also many influences on those taking decisions – not only advertising, evidence, anecdote, experience, consumer pressure but also national guidance and, it is hoped, the influence of local strategic medicines management. In this complex system it is hard to establish what changes result from intervening in a particular way. Previous chapters examine the core activities of strategic medicines management – the formulary, horizon scanning, critical appraisal and guideline development; this chapter looks at how these activities can be put together to approach medicine use in a systematic way. It examines how synthesis of the various elements might produce an impact that is bigger than the sum of its parts. In addition, the place of policies restricting access are considered, and the role of shared care guidelines. The approach that two organisations have taken to the overall medicines management system will be discussed. The two are chosen as 'case studies' because they have been described in the literature, not because they have shown to be the best performers.

A systematic approach

Taking a systematic approach to strategic medicines management is when an organisation or health community seeks to arrange structures, policies and practice in a deliberate attempt to make a real difference to the way medicines are used. Individual interventions such as formularies and guidelines play a part of this whole package. Most organisations probably set out to have systems that interlink and thus deliver the vision, but occasionally taking a step back and considering how well elements interlink can highlight the need for review and change. Various documents have, over the years, given prompts for this stocktaking process. *A Prescription for Improvement,* health circular HC (88) 54 and, for hospitals, *A Spoonful of Sugar* could each fall into this description.[1-3]

For there to be a well-organised, systematic approach, there should be a clear vision. 'Vision' tends to be a word that falls into disrepute; George Bush Senior dismissed it in a throwaway comment: 'the vision thing', when challenged over the need to look at the longer term, and it may be considered to be an excuse for substance.[4] However, in discussing effective organisations, Handy provides evidence that the success of organisations is in part dependent on the vision of their leaders, the ability to see the big picture.[5] For strategic medicines management, this means being clear about the purpose of activity. If it is about making the most of medicines, then the policies and practices need to support that. There are several contributing elements. These include: gaining resources for effective medicines to be accessible, investing in medicines that give the biggest benefits (assuming not everything is affordable), basing decisions and guidelines on evidence, then implementing these decisions and policies. These elements will support the overall vision.

Seeking to get the most from medicines may entail restricting access to some medicines in some circumstances. Failure to apply decisions can undermine the purpose and reduce credibility in the system used. Although achieving financial balance is a requirement of NHS organisations, it is not the sole purpose of medicines management. Delivering more benefits to patients should be the aim, not controlling spend, but failure to live within available resources will ultimately put patients at risk. The drive simply to control spend has often provided reason to examine an organisation's overall approach to strategic medicines management.

Examples from the literature

Although cited in Chapter 3 as a confounding factor while investigating the effect of a formulary on spend, the work Baker *et al.* reported as the broad approach to controlling spend could be seen as an early example of a systematised approach to strategic medicines management.[6] They reported changes of policy for outpatient supplies, reducing waste and improvements in purchasing practice alongside their revised formulary system. Several activities were initiated with the single aim of controlling spending on medicines.

The health circulars of 1988 also suggested a multifaceted

approach to good medicines use.[2] Hospital clinical pharmacy services, involvement of pharmacists in priority care groups in the community, DTC development, formularies and medicine use review were each included in the circular as important aspects of pharmaceutical services. The circulars gave an opportunity for pharmacy services to be reviewed and investment sought. Taken as a package, there was the basis of a systematic approach to medicines management.

In 1998, Fitzpatrick and Coker discussed the various aspects of strategic medicines management in their description of prescribing controls.[7] They listed the elements of these controls but pointed to the need for a whole system approach. Getting each element right was deemed essential, but the implication made was that this alone was not enough. Integration of the elements into a total package was proposed.

For secondary care the medicines management framework provided an assessment tool for these activities.[8] It drew out seven areas for action that, together, could be taken as a systematic approach to medicines management. The Audit Commission supported this systematic methodology, asking trusts to compare their own performance against the 19 recommendations for action included in *A Spoonful of Sugar* and proposing action plans be developed to bring performance to that of the best.[3]

The idea of a systematic approach to medicines management sounds laudable and the examples and documents mentioned so far put some flesh on the bones of the idea, but what does this approach mean in practice? To illustrate this, two examples of hospital trusts that have presented their approaches in the literature will be examined as case studies.

Southampton

Southampton University Hospitals NHS Trust reported work that they described as the optimising drug value project.[9] Their work began in 1997 and came as a response to financial pressures, in particular the problem of approving medicines on a 'scientific basis' but then having no funding to support their use. A report was developed, based on a series of interviews with clinicians and managers, aimed at identifying the perceived strengths and weaknesses in medicines management systems. Then an action plan to build on strengths was produced and investment made.

To increase the effectiveness of the already established clinical pharmacy service, therapeutic substitution was introduced. Pharmacists were empowered to make changes to inpatient medicine charts without the prospective agreement of the individual clinician. These were within agreed guidelines and undertaken by experienced members of the team. The changes each related to specific DTC decisions regarding choice of therapy. A second change for pharmacists was described as the advanced dispensing of discharge medicines; this was a system that allowed pharmacists to write up a discharge request based on the inpatient chart. Southampton reported that this change considerably reduced the time required to contact doctors regarding problems with discharge prescriptions. Both developments sought to use pharmacists' skills while controlling costs and improving safety.

A further change that fits into the description of medication management given in this book's introduction was made. A patients' own medicine scheme was established – using medicines brought into hospital by patients instead of dispensing new supplies, along the lines of other schemes already in the literature at that time. Waste was avoided and hospital costs were reduced, without an adverse impact on primary care.

Committee structures were reviewed, the trust DTC given a stronger role in monitoring finances and a new subcommittee was set up, called the drug finance group. This subgroup was given funds to administer on behalf of the DTC, seeking to invest in items given support on the basis of evidence and the expected health benefits. The DTC also had increased support from the medicines information department (a regional and local centre combined) who provided horizon scanning and trend analysis.

Another action included was a review of purchasing, embracing a parallel import partner and benchmarking on prices. Additional training for junior doctors on prescribing was developed. The hospital also set up a system of recording representative visits to the site. Additional pharmacists were appointed to lead the directorate pharmacist service and to provide support for junior clinical pharmacy staff.

Southampton made this series of changes in staffing, structures and policies to address medicines management issues. They reported a multi-faceted attempt to shift the organisation's culture to one where only affordable, evidence-based developments took place. Their report in *Hospital Pharmacist* claimed some success based on a slowing in growth of spending. They reported the difference in activity growth (measured in finished consultant episodes) and medicine spend growth. In the three years prior to the project, growth in spend on medicines was 8%, 13% and 8% above the growth in activity. In the first and second years of implementation, growth was 2.5% below activity and then 2.3% above activity, respectively. It is, however, very difficult to be certain of the impact that optimising drug value had on these figures. Case mix changes, outpatient activity changes and fortuitous price reductions may each have had an important effect. These years were also before NICE appraisals. Now, simply measuring growth in spend compared with growth in activity would have even less meaning – failing to increase expenditure could mean that NICE guidance is not being implemented.

Southampton reported that they had reasonable medicines management and clinical pharmacy systems in place, but they sought this multifaceted change to improve controls. The concept of making a number of small, specific changes together, to cause a significant shift, is one worth considering for medicines management and other change management projects.

North Staffordshire

The year following Southampton's description of their project to improve medicines management, work undertaken at the North Staffordshire hospital was shared in the *Pharmaceutical Journal*.[10] As at Southampton, the authors reported a long history of formulary use and other medicines management initiatives but they also noted four areas of concern that motivated them to initiate change. The four were:

- the ability for consultants to request non-formulary medicines for individual patients, leading to creeping developments
- the DTC having no means to fund the decisions that they took to permit new medicines
- senior management not aware of the cost pressures on the medicines budget
- no budget management system at directorate level.

It is interesting, although not surprising, that the same issue facing the DTC in Southampton emerged as a problem in North Staffordshire – no funds to back DTC decisions. No doubt this was common throughout the country. Pressure on primary and secondary care budgets has been continuous; the NICE technology appraisals have dealt with the funding issues in part, but not all medicines are covered and there still needs to be 'planning and managing'.

The overall response to North Staffordshire's four areas of concern was to revise the medicines management system. Four streams of work were developed:

- managed entry of new medicines
- pharmaceutical advice
- senior management information and attention
- purchasing pharmaceuticals.

As discussed in Chapter 3, formularies are often implemented as binding for junior staff but as guidance for consultants – or perhaps even as suggestions. North Staffordshire took this approach with a consultant signature required on non-formulary prescriptions. In 1997 an additional step was added: consultants were still permitted to request non-formulary medicines but had to seek support of their clinical director – the lead clinician for a directorate. A proforma was developed that was completed before the supply of the non-formulary medicine.

A DTC of sorts was developed as a group accountable to the executive board. It was called the Medicines Management Group and it supplemented other DTCs in the trust. It also had the remit of considering new, high-cost medicines. Unlike Southampton's drug finance group, it was not reported as having a delegated budget. However, it did approve medicines for use in two ways: where the trust had funds to support and where a business case seeking further funding was required. In the latter case the group assisted the development of that case. North Staffordshire reported rejecting 60% of the requests made for new, high-cost medicines, supporting 13% and seeking business cases for funds from the health authority for 25%. All cases in this final category were funded alongside the development of guidelines for use. This seems to be a successful approach to the controlled, self-managed introduction of new medicines. Importantly, the use of a guideline or protocol restricting or guiding access at the start of introduction can give confidence to the funders and prevent the overspill into usage that is either less cost-effective or has a weak evidence base. The NICE guidelines have this element, approved for use in x circumstance, not for use in y.

North Staffordshire had the benefit of working closely with a single health authority. Working with large numbers of commissioning organisations could be more problematic. The full impact of new funding streams in the NHS might deal with developments in a more standard way.

North Staffordshire also saw additional clinical pharmacy input to extend coverage to all medical wards. Delivering strategic medicines management without clinical pharmacy is likely to be frustrating and even could put patients at risk. Pharmacists working at an individual patient level can interpret and use the strategic medicines management framework without losing sight of the patient's individual needs. Pharmacists working at the next level up, with directorate teams, were used to support prescribing audit, cost-saving initiatives and guidelines. Clinical pharmacologist support for the directorate teams and work with the formulary pharmacist enabled structured reports on prescribing to be fed back to the clinical teams. Use of budget reports, reports on developing trends, and on individual prescribers' divergence from the agreed prescribing patterns have an important role. They can help the general and clinical managers in a directorate support the medicines management efforts. Feedback to individual prescribers can encourage reflective practice and even help apply peer pressure.

Board attention was brought to medicines issues by preparing quarterly reports, with figures and commentary so that an overview could be given. Financial and quality issues were included. Purchasing was improved by a closer working relationship between directorate pharmacists and the procurement team. The results of this multifaceted review were reported as a reduction in spending in year 1 and a slower growth than historically in place during year 2. The figures given were a fall in overall spend in 1998–99 of £0.5 million and a growth of only 5.6% in 1999–2000. This was a similar pattern to that reported by Southampton, although they had not claimed an absolute fall in expenditure. The results in each case are similar to the figures mentioned in Chapter 3 on the introduction of formularies – an initial impact then a slowed growth that suggests the benefits are retained.

The North Staffordshire authors argued that the success was dependent on the systematic approach taken. A raft of measures was used to build on an already reasonable system. Whether the Southampton, North Staffordshire or other models are used, organisations can reflect on the weaknesses of their current systems and develop action plans to improve their medicines management systems. The two models described here are secondary care based, but a parallel, multifaceted approach could be used across a health community or within a primary care organisation.

Shared care arrangements

It was difficult to decide where shared care guidelines fit in the structure of this book. They tend to support the 'traffic light' systems mentioned in the discussion of DTCs – indeed, they were recommended as part of the Midland Therapeutic Review and Advisory Committee (MTRAC) decisions. They have also been suggested within NICE guidance: riluzole, for example.[11] For convenience, shared care guidelines have found a home in this chapter on systematic approaches to medicines management, as they do support the move, in a controlled way, of complex or problematic medicines from secondary or tertiary care, to primary care. Shared care guidelines have also been described as shared care protocols. The former name will be used here.

In 2001, Duggan *et al.* reported their work evaluating shared care guidelines in the UK.[12] They noted the development of such guidelines from 1991, with cost shifting as a major motivator. As described in the opening chapter, until financial flows were unified, there was the opportunity to move prescribing costs to general practice to protect secondary care budgets. Developing shared care for financial reasons may have been expedient, but that does not seem to be a good basis for developing care.

In 1994, the executive letter on purchasing and prescribing highlighted the need for the provider units to ensure that local arrangements existed, on which hospital-led medicines ought not to be passed to GPs.[13] The letter also asked that arrangements be made for those medicines requiring special arrangements before being passed to GPs. A checklist also asked that these arrangements gave GPs appropriate information and support that enabled them to prescribe for and monitor patients. Following this, MTRAC was set up in 1995 in the West Midlands region to give advice and guidance on which medicines should be supported by shared care arrangements. Tacrolimus was one medicine included in this category.[14]

Although potentially helpful, shared care guidelines have been problematic. Reaching agreement at a local DTC on a shared care guideline, although important, is only one step in the process. Individual GPs may still not remain comfortable to take on the prescribing of specialist medicines where they lack the skills to take responsibility. Monitoring response and side-effects, and adjusting dosage may require knowledge seemingly straightforward to the specialist but beyond the usual experience of a GP. Biochemical results of tests undertaken in secondary care have not always been readily available to GPs when it is time to prescribe, although they retain professional responsibility and should only prescribe when they are assured it is safe to do so. Shared care guidelines do not replace the need for good communications between the specialist and the GP. Problems are guaranteed if they are used in this way.

Ashcroft *et al.* reported experiences of shared care arrangements for erythropoietin.[15] This was an early example of shared care, as the availability of this agent for renal units coincided with particular financial pressure on the NHS. They noted that 11 patients within their survey (total 119, 72% response) stated their GP had not been aware of the dose required at the point of prescribing, as dosage adjustments had been made in secondary care. However, they did comment that the shared care approach seemed to work.

The work by Duggan *et al.*, mentioned earlier, was a little more critical.[12] They undertook a survey and used content analysis to examine shared care guidelines. They noted that GPs were often excluded from the production of shared care guidelines and that the perception of their use as a cost-shifting device was described as a significant barrier to their use.

The area DTC could be an appropriate place to identify the need for a shared care guideline. Their use should be to support GPs to prescribe more complex therapies, where the patient can benefit from access to the medicine in primary care. This patient-centred rather than financed-focused approach is important. Placing prescribing in primary care can mean that additional trips to an acute hospital, possibly at some distance, are avoided. It can also mean that the GP has a better understanding of the healthcare for their patient. The approach also fits with the general principle of moving care from a tertiary/secondary setting to primary care, where this is safe and appropriate.

Shared care arrangements may be requested at the stage of appraising how a new medicine fits in to practice or later in a medicine's life cycle. General practitioner, specialist doctor, pharmacist and patient input into the shared care guideline can ensure that an appropriate document is developed. A clear statement of the responsibilities of each professional involved in the care is essential. Details of monitoring requirements and arrangements need to be included. There needs to be local agreement on how use of shared care guidelines fits in with the general medical service contract; some items needing particular monitoring are mentioned but others are not.

Once a suitable shared care guideline is in place it becomes the responsibility of the prescriber initiating therapy to ensure that the aspects of care taken up by the GP are handed over in a mutually acceptable way. Issuing a copy of the shared care guideline to support a letter requesting that care is shared may be the best approach. This may occur immediately when the patient commences therapy or after a period of stabilisation.

Figure 7.1 summarises the approach that can be taken in developing and using shared care guidelines. Reviewing individual arrangements and the general application of a guideline can allow modification or confirmation that it is working. The overriding principle should be what is best for the patient, although use of resources must not be overlooked. If this aspect of strategic medicines management is undertaken effectively,

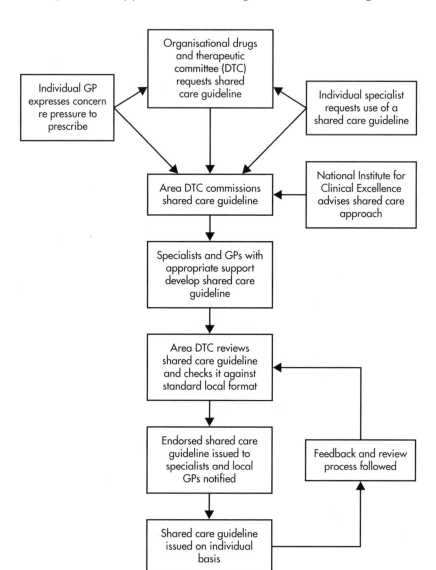

Figure 7.1 Developing and using shared care guidelines.

the risk of such arrangements being 'dumped prescribing orders' can be minimised and shared care guidelines can live up to their name.

Influencing prescribers

It could be argued that much of the work described by the term 'strategic medicines management' is about influencing those taking prescribing

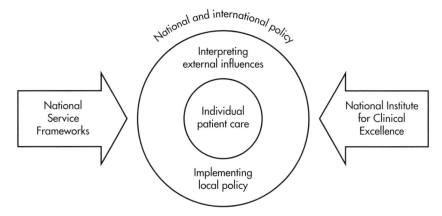

Figure 7.2 The place of strategic medicines management.

decisions. Figure 7.2 repeats Fig. I.3; it reminds us of the multilayered description of medicines management described in the introduction. Direct influence on prescribers in hospital is delivered by the clinical pharmacy team (clinical pharmacy is of course more than an influence on prescribers; direct care and support for patients, among other tasks, are covered by that term). Strategic medicines management is the next layer, and can be described as the indirect influence. Figure 7.3 attempts to identify the various layers. It describes a hospital system, but for primary care there are parallels, particularly if, in an extended team, an active part is played by the pharmacist providing the dispensed medicines.

Medicines information

Medicines information services play an important part in supporting medicines management at the individual and strategic level. The national network role played by UKMi is described in Chapter 4, leading on horizon scanning and preparing documents on emerging products. The UKMi website (www.ukmi.nhs.uk) and DrugInfoZone (www.druginfo-zone.org) are important sources of information and gateways to a range of resources that support strategic medicines management. Regional and local centres are the source of information and of critical appraisal skills, and can provide support by issuing various active medicines information bulletins. Primary care pharmacy teams may use medicines information support in preparing their own bulletins and documents.

This is just a mention of a few aspects of a vital service for strategic medicines managers. Prescribers, primary care lead pharmacists,

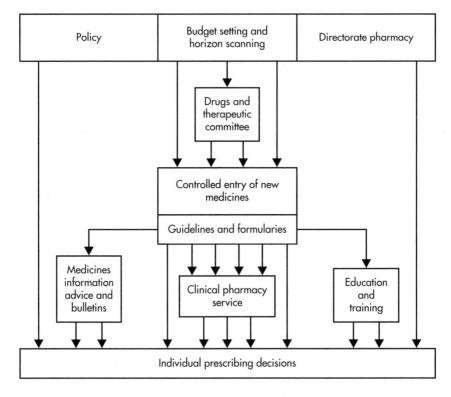

Figure 7.3 The multilayered nature of strategic medicines management.

hospital directorate and chief pharmacists and DTCs should all understand what medicines information can offer and use the resources to make the most of medicines.

Education and training

The medicines management framework for hospitals includes a section on influencing prescribers.[16] The emphasis is around the point of prescribing and this is important. Better to discuss the appropriate decision than to ring a junior doctor later to try to improve or correct the prescription. However, induction, education and training, and continuous professional development for prescribers provide important opportunities to influence. Induction for junior doctors should address safety as well as systems of strategic medicines management. Often there is little time in formal induction sessions to do more than point out where the pharmacy is and remind doctors how controlled drugs should be prescribed. Use of electronic learning packages and regular early contact in practice at ward level may be more effective in explaining how the local arrangements work. Consultants too require information on DTCs, formulary systems and the approach taken to guideline development. After induction, junior staff can be provided with advice and feedback on prescribing, and multiprofessional teams can learn from audit and clinical meetings. The possibly helpful, possibly disruptive learning that can form part of semi-promotional educational meetings for junior medical staff provided by the pharmaceutical industry are problematic. They will take place and a realistic approach is needed. Understanding the messages being given, and dealing with any changes in prescribing that result is the pragmatic way to respond.

The arrival of pharmacists as prescribers may be a positive influence on junior medical staff. Electronic prescribing systems can provide on-the-spot influence and serve as an educational tool.

In primary care, practice meetings, feedback to individuals on prescribing patterns and the process of developing guidelines can serve as educational tools. Meetings involving secondary care specialists and GPs provide educational and relationship building opportunities. Such meetings should support DTC-agreed practice and can be used to launch guidelines developed locally.

Directorate and practice pharmacists

In primary care, the practice is a natural unit for review of prescribing and other issues. In acute hospitals, directorates and divisions have been developed since the reforms in structure during the 1990s. The involvement of clinicians alongside general managers in running sections of a trust was the driver. Typically a directorate would encompass a group of wards of the same speciality: general surgery or elderly care medicine, plus the medical staff associated with the speciality. Divisions tend to be larger, grouping all medical specialities; all surgical specialities into single divisions would be the norm. The management team might include a nurse, a doctor and a general manager. In mental health trusts there may be similar management groupings: old-age psychiatry and adult psychiatry, for example, or care may be organised on a locality basis.

Whatever the specific nature of the arrangements, senior pharmacist advice focusing on medicines usage would be an important influence supplementing the clinical pharmacy service. Many have developed these arrangements with reports in the literature from the early 1990s.[17,18] The development of the role is a natural progression from that of the specialised clinical pharmacist, but not all specialised pharmacists wish to take on the broader semi-management role the directorate requires. A continued, direct patient-care role is a perfectly reasonable alternative. It will be interesting to see how this develops as the consultant pharmacist emerges.

Skills needed include an ability to work with prescribing data, whether hospital-computer generated or prescribing analysis and cost data (PACT) in primary care. An ability to present and persuade, using information, to negotiate and to plan is also essential. Clearly, a solid understanding of the medicines used and the clinical issues as well as aspects of policy will be needed. Personal credibility and interpersonal skills will enable the directorate or locality pharmacist to use their knowledge and medicines management skills to best effect.

Directorate, and other 'organisational unit', pharmacists can undertake audit, lead on or support guideline development, provide feedback on prescribing, help tailor horizon scanning, support the development of business cases for investment, assist in budget management and provide educational programmes. They may also take on broader roles in the directorate and continue with their underpinning clinical pharmacy work – whether running a clinic in general practice or involvement at ward level. These are potentially challenging and rewarding roles, vital in the delivery of high-quality, strategic medicines management.

Clinical audit

Clinical audit can be described as where the multiprofessional team examines clinical practice against pre-determined standards, with a view to learning lessons and implementing change. A detailed description of the way audit in healthcare has developed and how it can be implemented will not be addressed here, but audit has an important part to play in strategic medicines management systems. Examining if clinical guidelines are being implemented, including NICE guidelines, is a vital way for an organisation to check and improve performance. Feedback to prescribers and to those assisting good medicines use should help inform and educate.

Restricting access and saying 'no'

The formulary has been used in hospitals for many years to guide prescribing choices along pre-agreed, restricted paths. As discussed, the formulary is often binding for junior doctors but consultant staff are permitted to move outside the formulary, possible after some additional step, such as the North Staffordshire proforma. Others apply the document for all prescribers. The approach taken to restrict access to medicines tends to be by influence and negotiation rather than by application of policy – although there may be a set process to follow. Individual review and discussion of a non-formulary or new medicine may take place, and there is audit and expenditure monitoring. Where prescribing appears to be atypical it may be raised as a matter of performance under the remit of clinical governance. What about circumstances where prescribing moves or seeks to move outside the range of medicines supported by the local DTC when (a) the medicine is seen to offer no additional benefits at extra cost compared with a formulary medicine and (b) the medicine is newly available and has not been supported on the grounds of evidence or cost-effectiveness or affordability? These are situations, along with occasions where NICE has proposed restrictions on the use of medicines, where an organisation may wish to bind all prescribers to the DTC decision, not just junior hospital doctors.

The subject of restricting access to particular medicines is difficult – there are legal and ethical issues involved. A full discussion of all legal matters and the examples from case law goes beyond the scope of this book and this author, but a few key issues will be mentioned. The arrival of the blacklist and greylist in the 1980s restricted the prescribing of a range of branded medicines and of certain products seen as less beneficial, but generally GPs are seen as allowed to prescribe what they believe necessary for their patients. Newdick argues that paragraph 43 of the Terms of Service of GPs makes clear that 'any drugs . . . which are needed' shall be prescribed and that all necessary services should be provided.[19] Newdick was writing before the new general medical services contract, but a very similar paragraph (number 39 in part 3) to that quoted, regarding prescribing, is found in the revised document.[20] It could be argued that the thrust of the paragraph is to discuss how prescribing takes place rather than a statute dealing with access to all medicines but, taken with other aspects of the provision of service, Newdick presents a strong case to support a GP's duty to prescribe any medicines needed by their patient. (Paragraph 39 of the GMS contract states: 'Subject to paragraphs 42 and 43, a prescriber shall order any drugs, medicines or appliances which are needed for treatment of any patient who is receiving treatment under the contract by issuing to that patient a prescription form or a repeatable prescription and such a prescription for or repeatable prescription shall not be used in any other circumstances.') In terms of the controls on spending in primary care prescribing during the 1990s, he argues that seeking to discipline a doctor for prescribing required medicines that cause indicative prescribing limits to be exceeded would have been unlawful and quotes the government's own words at the time: 'It remains committed to ensuring that patients get the drugs that their doctors judge appropriate to their clinical needs.'[21] Newdick re-examined the issues in an article in 1998, following the NHS changes announced in 1997.[22] He noted the move to increase the involvement of GPs in the allocation of resources but restated the views on the duty to prescribe, although acknowledging there is an argument that restricting access to treatments may be inevitable.

Discussion and influence and a shared approach to rational prescribing, including involving patients in decision making, seem to be the necessary approach in primary care. Where spending exceeds funding owing to a few prescribers using more costly or non-approved medicines, peer challenge and sharing information, rather than issuing edicts, is the way forward.

What is the situation in secondary care? It is worth reflecting on the cases and comment drawn together by Ham and McIver as part of a series on policy dilemmas.[23] They explore five cases where decisions not to treat or to make a therapy available were contested. This was a continuation of the discussion that emerged from the Child B case where a decision not to treat was disputed.[24,25] Not all the five cases Ham and McIver discuss relate to medicines, but a case of access to Taxol (paclitaxel) and another regarding interferon beta for multiple sclerosis are included. In these two cases the patients' doctors did wish treatment to proceed (in a further case that was challenged, this was not so). These two are therefore pertinent to the discussion on restricting access; both cases related to funding restrictions. The interferon beta case was, however, complicated by the fact that government guidance had been issued; a failure of the health authority to take note of this guidance was an important factor in the decision not to fund being overturned at judicial review. The Taxol case did not get as far as judicial review. The public health advice of the health authority was to decline support for the therapy on the basis of newness and uncertainty of the evidence. This was challenged publicly, as the patient approached the local press. The opinion of a second oncologist was sought. On reviewing the case he commented that the patient was likely to respond to treatment and that toxicity was not a problem. Treatment was therefore funded.

One of the cases regarding medicines and other cases discussed by Ham and McIver involved judicial review.[23] Newdick comments that the courts are very careful about overruling the decisions made by health service managers regarding the use of resources.[19] He quotes Balcombe who ruled at appeal regarding access of a child to treatment, who stated the 'absolute undesirability of the court' to compel doctors or a health authority to make scarce resources available to one particular individual when others might gain more. However, Newdick also states that the courts will consider whether the decision maker allocating resources, refusing to support a treatment perhaps, has acted reasonably. Ham and McIver state that there is a well-established reluctance in English courts to rule against authorities who have decided not to fund a particular service or therapy.[23] However, where guidance has been ignored or a blanket decision taken that ignores the specifics of a case, a court will do so. The onus is on the decision maker to have a robust process of reaching a decision, then to have a mechanism for dealing with cases that may challenge that decision.

For strategic medicines management, the evidence-based appraisal process, supported by good horizon scanning and budget planning, must be the starting point for consideration of a policy that binds all prescribers and means that patients do not normally have access to a particular medicine. If these elements are not in place, then how could a trust claim to have a reasonable prioritisation process? Taking the line that no new medicine should be prescribed until NICE has supported it, is simply not good enough. If these elements are in place and a decision to refuse to support a medicine on the basis of cost-effectiveness or affordability is taken, albeit reluctantly, then a challenge via the courts may not be successful. A general policy of 'medicine x is not available' would also need an appeal or review mechanism for cases where the clinician or patient feels there is particular merit in the treatment in the specific circumstances. Hospital DTCs should consider preparation of explicit policies that have board understanding and backing. Policies should describe how access is restricted, the decision-making process and methods of appeal. Ideally, as has been described in earlier chapters, decisions should be jointly taken across the health community. These are not easy matters and run contrary to the way most healthcare staff wish to work, but as demand exceeds ability to respond, they must be faced. There has often been a focus on access to medicines – indeed, NICE was established in part to prevent variable access across England and Wales but, throughout the health service, decisions are taken each day that prioritise one service or intervention over another. Allowing all patients to have access to every conceivable medicine that may provide even a diminishingly small benefit, means that there is less resource for nursing staff numbers or wards, access to therapies or even the provision of counselling on how to make best use of the medicines prescribed.

Conclusion

The chapter considers the way in which a number of features of strategic medicines management can be put together to deliver rational, affordable and effective use of medicines. Health communities should seek to work together to achieve this systematic approach. Work evolving in Glasgow was reported in the *British Medical Journal* in 1998.[26] Beard *et al.* described their four-pronged approach: encouraging cost-effective prescribing, investing only in 'proved worth' medicines in hospitals, educating the public and joint working across the community. They sought to establish a drug evaluation unit to oversee this programme. These strands and the approaches discussed earlier can form the basis of a coherent local system.

Structures need to be in place – the DTCs. Policies and processes on how decisions will be taken, what restrictions can be placed, rights of appeal and so on should be established. These processes should gain the support of the executives and boards of individual organisations. Rapid, high-quality critical appraisal of evidence to inform decision making should be available, although use of national documents where available can avoid duplication of effort. Systems of induction, education and communication should be in place to support the medicines management process. Expert advice, supported by timely information should be available to the appropriate level of the organisation – practice, locality or directorate. A multiprofessional approach with public and patient involvement is required. The realities of financial constraints should be openly discussed and decisions taken to prioritise use of resources. Regular review of how the systems are working is advisable – North Staffordshire and Southampton felt they had reasonable medicines management, but both reported improvements following their reviews.

An aspect not addressed by either organisation was around risk to patients. Good use of medicines, advice to prescribers, guidelines and so on inevitably have elements related to risk reduction, but a systematic approach should also be considered, which addresses the risks of medicines as well as managing spend. *Building a Safer NHS* addresses a range of aspects relating to the risks of medicines; organisations need to use this as a tool to inform their medicines management processes.[27] Reporting systems, risk assessments, assessing the risks relating to new products, training and education, learning why things go wrong and building safer systems are just some of the building blocks for a safer service.

References

1. Audit Commission. *A Prescription for Improvement: Towards More Rational Prescribing in General Practice.* London: HMSO, 1994.
2. Department of Health. *The Way Forward for Hospital Pharmaceutical Services* HC 88(54). London: DH, 1988. Also WHC 88(66) (Wales) 1988 and 1988 (GEN) 32 for Scotland 1988.
3. Audit Commission. *A Spoonful of Sugar: Medicines Management in NHS Hospitals.* London: Audit Commission, 2001.
4. Bush G. In Knowles E, ed. *Oxford Concise Dictionary of Quotations*, 4th edn, Oxford: Oxford University Press, 2001.
5. Handy C. *Understanding Organisations*, 4th edn. London: Penguin, 1993.
6. Baker J, Lant A, Sutters C. Seventeen years' experience of a voluntarily based drug rationalisation programme in hospital. *Br Med J* 1988; 297: 465–469.
7. Fitzpatrick R, Coker N. In Panton R, Chapman S, eds. *Medicines Management.* London: BMJ Publishing Group and Pharmaceutical Press, 1998.
8. Department of Health. *The Performance Management of Medicines Management in NHS Hospitals.* London: DH, 2001.
9. Stephens M, Tomlin M, Mitchell R. Managing medicines: the optimising drug value approach. *Hosp Pharm* 2000; 7: 256–259.
10. Fitzpatrick R, Mucklow J, Fillingham D. A comprehensive system for managing medicines in secondary care. *Pharm J* 2001; 266: 585–588.
11. National Institute for Clinical Excellence. *Technology Appraisal No. 20: Riluzole (Rilutek) for Motor Neurone Disease.* London: NICE, 2001.
12. Duggan C, Beavon N, Bates I, Patel S. Shared care in the UK: failings of the past and lessons for the future. *Int J Pharm Pract* 2001; 9: 211–216.
13. Department of Health. *Executive Letter EL(94)72: Purchasing and Prescribing.* London: DH, 1994.
14. Blenkinsopp A, Clark W, Purves I, Fisher M. Getting research into practice. In Panton R, Chapman S, eds. *Medicines Management.* London: BMJ Publishing Group and Pharmaceutical Press, 1998: 133–153.
15. Ashcroft D, Clark C, Gorman S. Shared care: a study of patients' experiences with erythropoietin. *Int J Pharm Pract* 1998; 6: 145–149.
16. Department of Health. Medicines management in NHS Trusts: hospital medicines management framework. http://www.dh.gov.uk/PublicationsAndStatistics/ Publications/PublicationsPolicyAndGuidance/PublicationsPolicyAndGuidanceArticle/fs/en?CONTENT_ID=4072184&chk=RuVaBK (accessed 15 December 2004).
17. Ketley D, Godfrey B. Pharmacy and clinical directorates at Leicester Royal Infirmary. *Pharm J* 1992; 248: 588–589.
18. Barber N. Improving quality of drug use through hospital directorates. *Qual Health Care* 1993; 2: 3–4.

19. Newdick C. *Who Should We Treat? Law, Patients and Resources in the New NHS.* Oxford: Clarendon Press, 1996.

20. General Medical Services Contract. Prescribing and dispensing, paragraph 39. http://www.legislation.hmso.gov.uk/si/si2004/20040291.htm#38c (accessed 8 December 2004).

21. Anon. *Priority Setting in the NHS: The NHS Drug Budget, Government Response to the Second Report from the Health Committee 1993–94.* London: HMSO, 1994.

22. Newdick C. Primary care groups and the right to prescribe. *Br Med J* 1998; 317: 1361–1364.

23. Ham C, McIver S. *Contested Decisions: Priority Setting in the NHS.* London: King's Fund, 2000.

24. Regina versus Cambridge DHA, ex parte B, 2 All ER 129, 1995.

25. Ham C, Pickard S. *Tragic Choices in Health Care.* London: King's Fund, 1998.

26. Beard K, Forrester E, Lee A *et al.* Systems and strategies for managing the drugs budget in Glasgow. *Br Med J* 1998; 317: 1378–1381.

27. Department of Health. *Building a Safer NHS for Patients: Improving Medication Safety.* London: DH, 2004.

8

Managing medicines budgets

'Annual income twenty pounds, annual expenditure nineteen nineteen six, result happiness. Annual income twenty pounds, annual expenditure twenty pounds nought and six, result misery.'[1] These words placed into Mr Micawber's mouth by Dickens form the golden rule for budgeting of all kinds – don't spend more than you can afford. Having this as an aim for managing the medicines budget in primary and secondary care is not controversial; achieving it is rather difficult. *A Spoonful of Sugar* reported that a third of hospital trusts overspent their medicines budget by more than 10% in 2000–01.[2] A little caution is required here, as trusts were asked to state opening budget and outturn expenditure. Some trusts may have made in-year adjustments because of income or investment or service changes that were not reported. However, the overwhelming impression given was that budgets could not be balanced, with 10 trusts reporting budgets 25% overspent by year-end in 2000–01. Pressures on primary care spending are also significant, with above-inflation growth year on year.[3] Many aspects of strategic medicines management support budget control – restricting access to medicines, use of guidelines and of formularies. These systems help ensure that medicines are used well and attempt to reduce risks, but they have clear financial implications. This chapter concentrates on some of the direct issues related to medicines budget management. After a return to the subject of horizon scanning, the chapter divides into a secondary care focus and a primary care focus, as arrangements are rather different in each sector. The principles of planning ahead, monitoring, taking action when going off target and of gaining ownership of the issue by those able to incur spend, are universal.

Horizon scanning and planning

Chapter 4 discusses the information support available nationally in the area of horizon scanning. The work of the NPC and UKMi is vital in informing primary care and hospital trusts and the patch DTCs of expected developments; in particular, the *Prescribing Outlook* documents provide details of NICE appraisals that are due and of other expected developments, and includes information on the expected costs for a given population.[4,5] Scanning the NICE website for the expected release of technology appraisals can help develop the planning process. These national standards will need some local modelling; an understanding of the relevant catchment area for secondary/tertiary care will be vital. Typically a district general hospital will have a reasonably well-defined population for most of its services; the expected impact can then be calculated on that basis. A tertiary centre may have different populations depending on specialities – some services local, some across a whole strategic health authority or across a wider region. The calculation thus needs to be tailored for the particular appraisal. In calculating impact there needs to be a view on uptake: will all those presenting with a certain malignancy that is expected to have a new NICE-approved treatment wish to receive it? Experience of the local medical oncologists may help with this. For planning purposes, a view will need to be taken on the outcome of the SMC or NICE process – a simple 'use' or 'do not use' will not always result. Calculating the impact needs to take into account the likely limits to the treatment. For Scotland the decisions delegated to boards will also need to be predicted. Clearly, with these caveats, this is not a precise process: a 'best guess', or informed estimate, of expected developments and their impact is being established.

The next layer of possible developments is the new medicines not to be reviewed by NICE and perhaps the parallel in Scotland, decisions delegated to boards. Again the *Prescribing Outlook* documents can help, but local discussion with clinicians is invaluable. What medicines are in the late stages of trials? Are the doctors aware of new agents or new uses of established medicines that they may wish to employ? An impact assessment needs to be done for each of these and added to the NICE list.

The developments list that is produced should receive some peer review. Trusts would benefit from sharing their information with other trusts. It is also useful to have the list examined by PCT colleagues, as well as by strategic health authority advisers. Ideally, an area DTC view on the development list could be provided. The developments that have a major impact and will not receive NICE attention may also require prioritisation for local appraisal.

So far, comments have been centred on new medicines and new uses. There must also be a view taken on trends for established medicines. This may have an important element of activity growth, particularly for hospitals. Will there be 300 more cases for orthopaedic surgery next year? What are the medicine costs? For primary care organisations, the considerations will include items such as improving access to statins or the impact of population changes. The Department of Health's advice to PCTs in England in 2003 also highlighted the need to think about primary/secondary care interface issues when setting prescribing budgets. For example, re-aligning funding to support greater quantities of medicines at discharge may be necessary.[6] Further information on primary care spending growth can be obtained from the Prescription Pricing Authority's Prescribing Support Unit's website.[7]

The medicines approved by NICE or SMC, other new medicines and new uses, and growth in established medicines form the developments list. Against this can be set the expected move to generic drugs on patent loss, savings expected in secondary care from contracting arrangements and planned savings programmes. Once again these figures will be best guesses or estimates. Some allowance for slippage will be required – will there be early implementation before NICE releases its rules in June, or will that be resisted? Will patients start treatment at once? With all these factors taken into account, an expected required percentage growth can be estimated. For the way local delivery plans and service-level agreements currently work in England, this process needs to take place for secondary care from November to January. There will then be many iterations through to April. Estimations for primary care need to be ready for practice budget setting and, of course, for them to commission the secondary care activity.

Having gone through the process of estimating medicine-spend growth, there may still be an arbitrary figure provided, based on national expected figures. This does not mean that there is no point in making local calculations; it will be essential to know the risks on the medicines budget for the year ahead. Horizon scanning needs time to be done well. Organisations will need to find arrangements that suit their staffing and local structures. However, the core process is to understand what is happening in the current year, to use national documents and websites to predict likely events in the year ahead, to share with local partners, to involve local experts and to make best estimates of an unpredictable future.

Although not so much horizon scanning, it is worth mentioning the need to build into future years' budgets the impact of pressure not predicted for the current year. Setting a budget for the coming year based on extremely good horizon scanning, but basing the starting point on current budget rather than actual spend will lead to problems. Doing this in January/February for the financial year starting in April is in itself a risk, but using predicted outturn rather than starting budget is an improvement. Once again there are technical dangers to avoid – a NICE development that was funded and began in June needs the full-year effect built in for the following year. If, for a hospital, the full-year effect was generously provided from day 1, then that factor needs to be allowed for in budget planning. Difficult discussions can occur between commissioning bodies and trusts as to what has been covered in uplifts and what remains unfunded. This has become particularly important since the requirement for PCTs to fund NICE developments. The area DTC should be able to provide an expert overview of such matters, although in the author's experience, there is some reluctance to become too embroiled in the interorganisational exchanges that can ensue. In fact, this reluctance is understandable as, although the DTC role should not be divorced from financial issues, its main purpose ought to be centred around best use of medicines. That said, there have been reported examples of a collaborative approach to allocating development monies for NICE guidance. The Pharmaceutical Society conference in 2003 included a discussion of the Bristol, North Somerset and South Gloucestershire collaboration to form a NICE college to review needs, support issue and monitor use of funds.[8] Such arrangements should bring transparency and joint ownership of decisions.

Managing budgets in primary care

Primary care probably spend about a fifth of their budgets on prescribing and prescribing activity, a much higher figure than secondary and tertiary care. Getting budgets and expenditure control right is an important task. The opening chapter discusses the impact of fundholding and of the changes in financial flows. The latter means that the budget for primary care prescribing and for commissioning all other services is unified. The need to manage prescribing costs has become an even more important part of primary care organisations' responsibilities. Before this change, considerable effort in terms of predicting, monitoring and managing had been a feature of the health authority and primary care agenda. The Audit Commission's *A Prescription for Improvement* gave an impetus to taking rational prescribing seriously, suggesting a range of strategies to improve primary care prescribing, not just cost-related ones.[9] Various other initiatives, policy change, use of incentive schemes and so on have followed, bringing us to the current arrangements for budget setting and approaches to management.

Primary care prescribing costs have for a number of years been monitored closely in considerable detail. The Prescription Pricing Authority aggregates data on the medicines dispensed and provides data on usage and costs incurred. The detailed information is known as prescribing analysis and cost data (PACT data). These are available to practices and to PCTs; they have been used by pharmacy and medical advisers to identify issues of concern and opportunities for change. Frischer and Chapman describe how PACT data are used to undertake a variety of cost-related and quality-related monitoring and to review activity.[10] Individual GPs have PACT data returned on a monthly basis. Use of electronic returns is being developed. On an organisational basis, electronic data are the norm. The Prescription Pricing Authority has developed ePACT.net as an access point where up to three years' data can be viewed and used to compare practices within the organisation. GPs prescribing at above average costs in a particular *British National Formulary* section can be highlighted and investigated. Higher-than-average spend on a group could be good or bad; high use of steroid inhalers may indicate that the balance of preventer-to-symptom relief is right. High spend on lipid-lowering agents may mean good application of the NSF; this needs more than a cursory look – more costly statins rather than generic statin may be driving up spend so that the number of patients treated is actually lower than a less costly practice. Kendall suggests that poor or inappropriate prescribing might be picked up via ePACT.net – citing the Shipman case and the potential for growth hormone misuse.[11] In Chapter 9 the performance management of medicines management is explored; PACT data are part of this process, with specific indicators feeding into the star rating systems for PCTs in England.

PCTs are not left in isolation to deal with prescribing costs. The Prescribing Support Unit has been set up by the Department of Health to undertake a number of tasks to improve primary care medicines. The unit's aims are:

- to provide analysis for the department in support of policy initiatives, particularly those related to cost-effective prescribing
- to support prescribing initiatives throughout the service by disseminating information
- to support researchers who are working in the field of prescribing.

The unit was also jointly responsible, with York University Health Economics Centre, for the pre-1999–2000 allocation formula for health authority's prescribing funds. The unit's website explains their current work as moving away from simply monitoring budget performance towards quality-related issues. These include working with the Prescription Pricing Authority to ensure that clinical governance is a 'team sport rather than a top down process.'[7] Developing indicators and toolkits to support prescribers is central in these efforts. Indicators have been around since the Audit Commission's report in 1994, with a revised set available in 1997. The Prescribing Support Unit's work on further indicators is now overseen by the Prescribing Indicators National Group, who have set standards for these indicators and aim to ensure that they are relevant and important to clinicians, available from naturally collected data and subject to change that is in the control of the doctor.

The first stage in managing any budget is to plan and agree it. In England, PCT funds are defined in the *Primary Care Trust Resource Limits* Health Service Circular that provides details for the three-year period commencing 2003–04.[12] Over this period growth in excess of 9% is available. PCTs must then decide the total budget for each year for prescribing and, in turn, set the individual practice prescribing budgets. Further guidance from the Department of Health is available *Primary Care Prescribing and Budget-setting 2003/04–2005/06*.[6] Guidance includes not only noting the planning priorities laid down by the department but also opportunities to make efficiency savings. As mentioned in the horizon-scanning discussions, primary care organisations must account for NSF implementation, NICE guidance, newly developed medicines and interface issues with secondary care. Individual practice budget setting is at the discretion of each PCT, historical spend with allowance for change being the typical approach. The Prescribing Support Unit can support this process and provides a budget-setting utility accessed via the website: www.psu.ppa.nhs.uk.

Once budgets are set, in-year monitoring and taking action to manage can be undertaken. The unit provides regular comparative data to enable practices and PCTs examine their own expenditure trends. Unlike secondary care, there has been much work done to allow inter-practice/organisation comparison. Basic measures such as items dispensed per patient, cost per patient and cost per item have been supplemented by more sophisticated indicators. In the early 1980s the first weighting factor was developed – the prescribing unit (PU). This attempted to allow for the greater need to use medicines among the over 65s. Rather than look at spend per patient as a measure to compare practices, spend per PU could be used. Each patient over 65 counted as 3 PU, each patient under that age as 1 PU. In 1993, the age, sex and temporary-resident-originated prescribing unit was developed (ASTRO-PU). This has nine different weightings – based on the factors listed in the title. Further development of therapeutic group measures has also taken place (specific therapeutic group age/sex-related-prescribing units, STAR-PU). There is an argument that simply looking at age and sex issues misses an important feature related to prescribing, that of social deprivation. Comparing practices that have very different socio-economic settings, merely by cost per ASTRO-PU, is seen as misleading. A Low Income Scheme Index has been developed to provide some help with this.

In addition to the major interventions described in this text (formulary, guidelines, DTC advice), a range of activities have been undertaken to manage prescribing budgets in primary care. Review meetings with pharmacy advisers based in health authorities during the 1980s and 1990s with PACT feedback and development of indicative prescribing budgets were some of the first active interventions. Prescribing incentive schemes were also introduced in many health authorities for non-fundholding practices. Such schemes were given a mixed reception but one observational study suggested that the introduction of financial incentives could produce changes in prescribing patterns.[13] It has been noted that these schemes and fundholding tends to have more impact on choice of medicine than they do on the decision whether to prescribe.[14] This is an interesting issue, of obvious relevance in considering use of antibiotics, of night sedation and other medicines; it returns to the Chief Medical Officer's letter in the *British Medical Journal* of 1980, which pointed out that the key question is: 'Should I write a prescription at all?' rather than which is the most economical medicine to prescribe.[15]

Prescribing incentive schemes were revisited in 1999 with the formation of primary care groups, later to evolve or to be transformed into PCTs. Indicators used to calculate payment included cost and quality measures. Ashworth *et al.* reported their use in London and the southeast but noted that rewards were not clearly connected to cost or quality improvements.[16] Cantrill reported work from the Tracker survey of English primary care organisations: 11 of the 57 responders had linked their incentive schemes to budget balance, 38 had linked incentives to generic prescribing rates and 34 to reduced antibiotic usage.[17] The final measure neatly linked cost and quality into one aspect of prescribing.

The Audit Commission health bulletin on prescribing in 2003 noted the impact of NSFs and that prescribing costs were outstripping funded growth, but they also commented that improved prescribing and the use of medicines management initiatives could take significant costs out in future years.[18] The Prescribing Support Unit toolkit identifies some of the areas where the Audit Commission state savings can be achieved. None are particularly surprising and have been part of advisers' agendas for many years: generic prescribing rates, avoiding medicines of limited clinical value, minimising to appropriate levels the use of premium-priced, modified-release preparations and combination products and reducing use of benzodiazepines.[19] Additionally, optimising cost-effectiveness in choice of steroid inhaler is an Audit Commission-led indicator.

The NPC guide for PCTs published in 2003 stresses the need for strong local strategies that take this work further. They should control spend but also ensure that resources are used to gain the health benefits associated with good prescribing.[20] Practice-based pharmacist advice to support rational prescribing, in addition to any direct pharmaceutical care provided, is likely to be a key part of the strategy. Use of community pharmacists to support local prescribing strategies may also be valuable. Leach *et al.* reported work in Dudley that enabled local community pharmacists to make interventions regarding strength of product optimisation (described as dosage efficiency), prescription length optimisation (attempting synchronicity in supplies) and use of generics.[21] Significant savings were reported and these ideas have been employed in medicines management collaborative work. The *Pharmaceutical Journal* had also reported a scheme from Hayes and Harlington where payment to pharmacists was made for interventions made.[22] Modernisation of the community pharmacy contract and changes suggested in *A Vision for Pharmacy* should enable the contribution from these frontline pharmacists to be increased.[23] This is a key area for medicines management at an individual level as well as in the context of this book's theme.

Repeat prescribing is an area where pharmacist input is being developed and has quality and cost implications. Repeat prescribing has been a focus in medicines management collaboratives in primary care and is the subject of an NPC guide that has British Medical Association and Royal College of General Practitioner support.[24] The good practice guide *Saving Time, Helping Patients* points out the high volume of prescribing that occurs on a repeat basis and the potential for waste. Getting this aspect of service right should help budget management but has a greater potential in terms of quality of care.

Part of the repeat-prescribing agenda must be to avoid waste. Prescribing and dispensing medicines which are duly collected but then stored in cupboards in patients' homes will bring no benefits but incur significant cost. Most healthcare professionals can recount anecdotal experience of patients with hoards of tablets they have regularly obtained but never used. To avoid this, or at least minimise the problem, patients need to be engaged in the decision-making process about their medicines. They should be encouraged to be open about which medicines they find helpful, and each member of the healthcare team needs to be looking out for difficulties in concordance. There is unlikely to be 'one best way' to achieve high levels of concordance, as we all vary in our attitudes to medicines and have differing abilities to cope with regimens, but this is a crucial part of good use of resources.

The focus so far has been on the English PCT, but the pressures and methods of control are common to all UK countries. In Wales, the All Wales Prescribing Advisory Group has updated a set of indicators for use by Local Health Boards.[25] These indicators build on those previously available, produced by the All Wales Medicine Strategy Group. An example of a cost-related indicator is the target of having simvastatin, the first statin to come off patent, at 45% or more of all the statin prescribing. Each board was also to have a formulary, produced in conjunction with their local secondary care provider.

The issue of new medicines in Scotland is discussed in Chapter 1. Much work takes place at local level with national support. The 1999 report of the Accounts Commission (an independent statutory body in Scotland supporting good use of resources) described the rapid growth in spend despite best efforts to control it.[26] The areas for action described were, not surprisingly, similar to those in the other UK countries. Organisational arrangements, PCTs and local healthcare cooperatives were described as providing opportunities for improving working arrangements; a total of £26 million a year savings were suggested as a target. The update provided in 2003 reported significant progress, with rises in generic prescribing and falling spend on medicines of limited value.[27] Further action to ensure that the most cost-effective agent gets chosen as first line by GPs, to improve repeat prescription systems and to develop national indicators, was proposed.

The strategic medicines management agenda for primary care organisations includes financial planning and control. There are twin responsibilities, first managing general practice and other primary care prescribing expenditure and, second, commissioning secondary and tertiary care services with a strong element of planning for developments in medicines use. Both areas require a multiprofessional team approach. The growing range of professionals who can prescribe, and the developments in 'out-of-hours' arrangements and walk-in centres, increase the complexity of the task. Appropriate local arrangements need to be in place for doctors, nurses, pharmacists, finance and general managers and others, to work successfully on planning and managing resources to support effective primary care prescribing.

Managing budgets in secondary care

In the *Textbook of Hospital Pharmacy*, Ross includes a paragraph on the medical budget.[28] He describes the need to consider spend on medicines and notes the arrival of computer systems. An alternative approach is suggested for those without such systems, whereby 'the costs of a sample of supplies can be calculated and used as a basis for the apportionment of total expenditure'. Since 1980, when this was first published, a very considerable change has occurred in the way medicine spend is monitored and managed. Computer systems for stock control, dispensing and distribution of medicines are now universal, with developments reported soon after the *Textbook*.[29] Today, the development is towards computerised prescribing systems, with electronically recorded nurse administration included. The opportunity this can bring regarding costing and management information should be as big a leap as the first stock systems, the move from ward-based costing to consultant team-based costs allowing hospitals to catch up with the level of detail so long available in primary care. The realisation that this gap causes a problem nationally as well as locally came to the fore in the 2004 reporting of uptake of NICE cancer medicines.[30] Data were available on hospital spend only from a third party who purchases hospital-spending figures. An impetus to bring forward e-prescribing resulted.

At a local level, responsibility for the medicines budget tended to rest centrally until the development of the directorate structure. The chief pharmacist was often the budget holder. The increased involvement of general management in the 1980s, the resource management initiatives and the return to greater clinical involvement in hospital management in the 1990s resulted in a move to devolve budgets to units within the hospital – the directorate or division. Accountability for the budget was intended to gain ownership and better control. Managing a series of budgets to 'the bottom line' could enable the directorate to invest savings made in prescribing into staffing or new developments. However, pressure owing to activity increase, new medicines and increased complexity plus the ever-present cost improvement or savings programme has meant the Micawber state of happiness tends to be rare. The system of a devolved budget where responsibility lies with the teams using the medicines appears preferable to a central purse from which everyone spends. That said, it remains important for the chief pharmacist and the trust DTC to keep an overview on expenditure and to play their parts in control. Best purchasing practice, avoiding waste and good strategic medicines management support are required for directorates to perform well.

An area of tension regarding budget responsibility is where one clinician prescribes or advises but the costs fall elsewhere. An anaesthetist prescribing a pre-operative medicine on a surgical ward, where the anaesthetist is not in that directorate, can lead to an argument over costs. Similarly a microbiologist prescribing or advising on anti-infectives without being too concerned about cost could lead to disengagement of the clinicians in the paying directorate. Computerised prescribing systems could link the prescriber to their own budget to overcome this. Devolving a budget for selected antibiotics or antifungals to the microbiology team may be an option even without computerised prescribing. However, a team approach to the issue of budget management, as it would be for clinical care in effective audit meetings, is probably a more mature approach even if it is harder to achieve.

The idea of the unusual or one-off prescribing need is worth considering. Should a devolved budget cope with all eventualities, or would a reserve for high-cost, unforeseen treatments be useful? The answer depends on the frequency and size of the problem. If most directorates have regular, although not predictable, requests then a reserve could be devolved along with the rest of the budget. If there is a more variable pattern, disproportionately affecting some directorates in some years, there may be merit in holding a centrally administered reserve for the costly unexpected requests. The system should not be a means of allowing creeping, otherwise unfunded, developments.

Information on spending on medicines is derived from the pharmacy stock control system or, more latterly, the computerised prescribing system linked in to the pharmacy system. Use of hospital versions of prescriptions that can be dispensed in the community (formerly the FP10HP) will not be captured in this way. Historically, after a long delay, the forms have been returned from the Prescription Pricing Authority along with a financial summary and a detailed paper version of the costs of items dispensed. These could be used to monitor trends and the costs devolved to prescribers. However, often the subdivisions used have been fairly broad. Sometimes a single code was shared between directorates. Even where more fitting groups were used, the delay and non-electronic nature of feedback made active management difficult, particularly important for community trusts and other services where prescribing was based across diffuse centres with no option of hospital pharmacy supplies to outpatients. Fortunately, steps have been taken to move to a system more akin to primary care. Pre-printed, coded prescriptions are available and data are available sooner and electronically. This electronic system became the standard approach in 2004.

Usually the budget statements received via the trusts finance system will provide only a few lines on the medicines budget, the pharmacy information team or directorate pharmacist providing more detail. Fitzpatrick reports the type of information that can be fed back to clinicians, budget managers and the board.[31] This needs to be accurate, timely and relevant. Preparing figures on the top 10 or 20 medicines, the items seeing most growth, and items recently introduced, may be particularly helpful. Linking these data to activity figures, and providing some commentary, can ensure that data become information to inform action. The board and the DTC will wish to see the key facts and trends; this becomes particularly important when budgets begin to be exceeded. DTCs within a trust and the area DTC could gain insight into their own performance by receiving data on the spending patterns where they have taken decisions or made investment. Knowing that an investment in a NICE therapy is being spent appropriately will give assurance; seeing that it is not, can lead to a complaint or concern being raised.

The issues of performance management are discussed in Chapter 9. However, it is worth noting that merely monitoring a budget is not sufficient; action needs to follow where expected performance is not being achieved. For a hospital's medicines budget this will mean seeking investment, imposing controls, achieving other savings, making virements or obtaining permission to overspend. The assumption made here is that the only direction of problem is an overspend – although underspending is the Dickensian happy state, it could be that benefits are not being gained and that expected developments are not implemented. Although a comprehensive literature review was not undertaken, the author did not find articles complaining of the problems of an underspending hospital medicines budget.

The options given to correct an overspending budget included seeking investment. Where additional activity has been provided there may be additional income to the trust. This should be reflected in the medicines budget. Reserves held to support in-year developments, such as in Southampton, may also be a source of investment.[32] PCTs will probably not be in a position to make investments in-year, as these should be addressed in the annual local delivery planning process. Certain high-cost medicines have sometimes been an exception.

Delaying the introduction of new medicines, where no NICE appraisal has been produced, may be one of the controls to bring an overspend into balance. Review of the medicines that contribute most to the spend – based on the author's experience, a small number of medicines produce half the spend – to check that their use is in line with guidance may also help. The remedies of earlier years – cost shifting to primary care – should not be contemplated. Writing to GPs to take on prescribing not affordable in secondary care is also unhelpful and likely to lead to conflict that can cause a loss of the patient's confidence in both parties. Where there are widespread spending problems in a trust, the systematic review discussed in Chapter 7 may be required. For a directorate or division, the option to switch budget from staff or equipment to support medicines spend may exist. This may be easy if a new medicine releases other costs, such as reducing nursing time or shortening length of stay. However, it may be hard to extract these costs even if the logic is correct.

Clear accountability and ownership, good information systems and willingness to act, all play important roles in delivering budget control in secondary care. Although information has been traditionally less well-developed than in primary care, there may be more levers for ensuring control.

Payment by results

An important change being brought into the NHS is a revision in the way that funds move between primary and secondary care to pay for services. *Reforming NHS Financial Flows, Introducing Payment by Results* was published in October 2002 by the Department of Health. It explained the intended move towards nationally agreed prices for specific aspects of care, beginning with elective care but extending to all commissioning arrangements.[33] The argument put forward was that, in the context of significant investment and improvement, a transparent and fair pricing system was needed for all providers, including in the independent sector, and that transaction costs could themselves be reduced by removing the argument over pricing between PCTs and trusts. Section 2.2 of *Reforming NHS Financial Flows* described the plan eventually to extend the scheme to GP-enhanced and additional services.

The payment scheme, for inpatient and day-case activity, is based on using a national average price for each healthcare resource group (HRG). An HRG is an intervention or group of interventions within a speciality that consume the same, or around the same, resource – they are described as 'iso-resource'. Initially 15 HRGs were included in the system, the first step of the phasing-in process during 2002–03. Examples of HRGs included are:

- cataract extraction, with lens implant
- coronary bypass
- percutaneous transluminal coronary angioplasty
- primary hip replacement
- bilateral hip replacement.

The price paid for these HRGs was derived from the national average price, or national tariff. This in itself is made up from the reference costs submitted by each NHS trust and includes clinical costs (theatre costs, medicines, medical and nursing time, and so on) and non-clinical costs (food, cleaning, management, capital charges). Allowance is made for long-stay patients and work on admission or assessment wards. Other details regarding market forces, 'unclassified' HRG codes are also addressed. Critical-care elements are reported separately from the main reference costs of HRGs and commissioned on a bed-day basis.

Payment by Results: Core Tools 2004 updated progress on the new system and included details of reference costs and tariff prices.[34] The range of reference costs remained large, an index-based system including all activity undertaken by each trust with the mean at 100; individual organisations have indices more than 25% above and others 25% below the mean. Clearly there are potential risks of moving towards the standard tariff for those trusts so far above the fixed price. Similarly PCTs whose providers are well below tariff will need to increase payment for the same level of work. A three-year transition from April 2005 was described in the 2004 document (subsequently there has been a delay in the process, with only elective services included for 2004–05). For 2004–05, 48 specific HRGs are covered by national tariff prices, increases and reductions in work done by trusts funded or refunded at national tariff rate. First-wave NHS foundation trusts were permitted to move one year ahead of the remaining NHS trusts. Outpatient episodes and other services such as ward attendees and chemotherapy medicine costs are also listed in schedules within the tariffs. The plan was to include outpatients in the system by 2005–06.

The revised system has the potential to make significant impact on financial flows throughout the NHS. There will be an effect on medicines management, as on all services, but a key question of relevance is how the tariff will take account of NICE and other developments. The department's question and answer response states: The [tariff] inflation uplift for 2003/04 includes an uplift to cover the cost of new technologies such as drugs, but there was no adjustment to the relative weights for individual HRGs to take account of differential effects of technology changes ... the 30–45 HRGs used for cost per case commissioning in 2004–05 will be reviewed to take into account the implications of NICE guidance.'[35] Some allowance, but not targeted allowance, is thus described.

A technical paper, 'to assist thinking not provide guidance', prepared in July 2003, discussed the funding of new technologies under 'payment by results'.[36] The paper notes that the payment at national tariff rate combined with the ability to retain surplus provides an incentive to reduce costs but a risk that new technologies do not receive investment. A number of counter-drivers are described: patient choice – a new system for patients with long waits to be able to choose where they receive treatments (the 'natural' meaning of the phrase is implied), professional pride, NICE, national inspection systems, performance management systems. International experience of similar systems is drawn upon and the conclusion made that a general inflation uplift should be provided plus an element of specific HRG adjustment where a significant impact is made by a piece of NICE guidance. Ideas such as holding a reserve at PCT level to be passed on once NICE guidance is implemented were suggested and further work was promised. The 2004 *Payment by Results* paper identified a composite uplift of 11.2% for the period 2003–05.[34]

Further guidance emerged in December 2004 with the arrival of *Implementing Payment by Results*.[37] The document explained that 'chemotherapy' (understood to mean cancer treatments including cytotoxic chemotherapy) was a service excluded from the general tariff system, and that there was a list of excluded medicines. Exclusions included: AIDS/HIV antiretrovirals, antitumour necrosis factors, interferon beta, hepatitis C therapy, riluzole, enzyme replacement therapies, photodynamic therapy and several others. For excluded medicines and excluded services a locally priced cost and volume agreement would need to be agreed. Presumably, an agreed baseline, then payment for each additional case would be established and used. The paper also noted a 'quality and reform' uplift that should account for changes in medicines, plus some specific adjustments to selected Health Resource Groups where there had been significant cost implications from guidance. An example in the paper was of glycoprotein IIa/IIIb costs being added to coronary care unit tariff rate. The guidance also referred again to pass-through payments, where a PCT could decide locally on specific uplifts to support new technologies.

These changes will not remove the need to scan and plan for developments, neither will they mean cost control and budget planning are redundant. In the transition years, organisations with high index costs will experience particular pressures to reduce costs. This will inevitably mean an examination of medicines management services and medicines use. It may be opportune for those organisations to undergo a review along the lines of that described in Chapter 7 in North Staffordshire or Southampton.

Conclusion

It is neither wise nor feasible to divorce managing the spend on medicines from other aspects of strategic medicines management. This chapter focuses on some of the mechanics of budget management and some of the strategies adopted to control spend not discussed elsewhere. A key feature discussed earlier is the potential waste of resources that prescribing unwanted medicines can cause. All organisations, but especially those in primary care, need to have a significant strand of their medicines management programme that concentrates on communication with patients and the public regarding telling their doctor or pharmacist about medicines no longer wanted. Prescribing cost-effective medicines that are taken, that bring real benefits and fit in with health priorities, underpins managing medicine budgets. Planning for developments, obtaining the funds needed and living within them are the key elements of medicine budget management.

References

1. Dickens C. Chapter 11. *David Copperfield*. First published 1850.
2. Audit Commission. *A Spoonful of Sugar: Medicines Management in NHS Hospitals*. London: Audit Commission, 2001.
3. Department of Health. *Statistical Bulletin 2003/12: Prescriptions Dispensed in the Community Statistics 1999–2002, England*. London: DH, 2003.
4. Davis H (ed.). *Prescribing Outlook – August 2003 Part A*. UKMi and NPC, 2003.
5. Sennik D, Erskine D. *Prescribing Outlook – October 2003, Part B*. London: UKMi, 2003.
6. Department of Health. *Primary Care Prescribing and Budget-setting 2003/04–2005/06*. London: DH, 2003.
7. Prescribing Support Unit. http://www.psu.ppa.nhs.uk (available to NHSnet users; accessed 31 May 2004).
8. Anon. Collaboration to allocate funds for NICE guidance. *Pharm J* 2003; 271: 415.

9. Audit Commission. *A Prescription for Improvement: Towards More Rational Prescribing in General Practice.* London: HMSO, 1994.

10. Frischer M, Chapman S. Issues and direction in prescribing analysis. In Panton R, Chapman S, eds. *Medicines Management.* London: BMJ Publishing Group and Pharmaceutical Press, 1998.

11. Kendall H. Why prescribing data are monitored. *Pharm J* 2004; 272: 21–22.

12. Department of Health. *Primary Care Trust Revenue Resource Limits 2003/4, 2004/5 and 2005/6.* HSC 2002/12. London: DH, 2002.

13. Bateman D, Campbell M, Donaldson L *et al.* A prescribing incentive scheme for non-fundholding general practices: an observational study. *Br Med J* 1996; 313: 535–538.

14. Bradley C. A primary care perspective on medicines management. In Panton R, Chapman S, eds. *Medicines Management.* London: BMJ Publishing Group and Pharmaceutical Press, 1998.

15. Yellowlees H. Cutting the drug bill (letter). *Br Med J* 1980; 280: 797.

16. Ashworth M, Golding S, Shepherd L, Majeed A. Prescribing incentive schemes in two NHS regions: cross sectional survey. *Br Med J* 2002; 324: 1187–1188.

17. Cantrill J. Prescribing incentives and guidelines. *Primary Care Pharm* 2001; 2: 1–3.

18. Anon. NSFs are driving prescribing costs to outstrip primary care budget increases. *Pharm J* 2003; 270: 465.

19. Prescribing Support Unit. Toolkit. http://www.psu.ppa.nhs.uk/pdf2003 _toolkit_info.pdf (available to NHSnet users; accessed 31 May 2004).

20. National Prescribing Centre. *PCT Responsibilities Around Prescribing and Medicines Management.* Liverpool: NPC, 2003.

21. Leach R, Hipkiss I, Hesslewood J. *et al.* Investigation into the effectiveness of the Dudley prescribing efficiency scheme. *Pharm J* 2003; 270: 276–277.

22. Anon. PCG pays pharmacists for prescription intervention. *Pharm J* 2000; 264: 5.

23. Department of Health. *A Vision for Pharmacy in the New NHS.* London: DH 2003.

24. National Prescribing Centre. *Saving Time, Helping Patients: a Good Practice Guide to Quality Repeat Prescribing.* Liverpool: NPC, 2000.

25. NHS Wales. High level prescribing indicators. http://www.wales.nhs.uk/sites/ documents/371/highlevelindicators%20ammended.pdf (accessed 8 December 2004).

26. Accounts Commission for Scotland. Supporting prescribing in general practice. http://www.accounts-commission.gov.uk/publications/pdf/1999/99hs_06.pdf (accessed 8 December 2004).

27. Audit Scotland. Supporting prescribing in general practice, a progress report, June 2003. http://www.accounts-commission.gov.uk/publications/pdf/ 2003/03pf04ags.pdf (accessed 8 December 2004).

28. Ross A. The area. In Allwood M, Fell J, eds. *Textbook of Hospital Pharmacy.* Oxford: Blackwell, 1980.

29. Hughes I. Computer systems in pharmacy: II. *Br J Pharm Pract* 1992; 4: 15–24.

30.   Department of Health. Cancer medicines uptake. http://www.dh.gov.uk/
       PublicationsandStatistics/Publications/PublicationsPolicyAndGuidance/
       PublicationsPolicyAndGuidancearticle/fs/en?CONTENT_ID=4083901&chk
       =vkfy2d (accessed 16 June 2004).
31.   Fitzpatrick R. Strategic medicines management. In Stephens M, ed. *Hospital
       Pharmacy*. London: Pharmaceutical Press, 2003.
32.   Stephens M. Economic analyses to assist drug entry decision making. *Pharm
       Manage* 2001; 17: 36–40.
33.   Department of Health. *Reforming NHS Financial Flows, Introducing
       Payment by Results*. London: DH, 2002.
34.   Department of Health. *Payment by Results: Core Tools 2004*. London: DH,
       2004.
35.   Department   of   Health.   http://www.dh.gov.uk/policyandguidance/
       organisationPolicy/FinanceAndPlanning/NHSFinancialReforms/
       NHSFinancialReformsArticle/fs/en?CONTENT_ID=400870&chk=2w2C14
       (now unavailable).
36.   Department of Health. *Payment by Results: Technical Papers, July 2003,
       Implementing Payment by Results and Investment in Technology and Drugs*.
       London: DH, 2003.
37.   Department of Health. *Implementing Payment by Results: Technical
       Guidance 2005/6, December 2004*. London: DH, 2004.

9

Performance management

Strategic medicines management has been described and its elements examined. This chapter discusses the performance management of strategic medicines management. But what is performance management? The definition that has been used elsewhere is offered here: performance management is the overarching process through which organisations achieved desired outcomes.[1] Performance management of individuals is also important and in itself contributes to achieving organisational aims. This includes dealing with poor performance, setting objectives, providing training and development, and giving feedback. However, here the focus will be on performance management above that individual level.

It could be argued that, for strategic medicines management, performance management should deal with health communities and not simply individual organisations. It is how the whole community deals with the entry of new medicines, communicates across organisational boundaries and so on, that is important. It is not just whether a PCT or a hospital achieves its own goals. However, because accountability is an important feature of performance management, the inevitable boundaries between organisations could make performance management of a health community rather difficult. It is probably best to accept that performance management will be undertaken for each individual organisation, but ensure that targets reflect the shared nature of strategic medicines management. Thus, each organisation should have 'desired outcomes' that benefit the community as a whole. Targets that demonstrate 'being a good partner' would be included. For example, a PCT may seek to ensure that 100% of practices can access locally agreed shared care guidelines; a hospital may have a target that 100% of letters to GPs where non-formulary medicines are recommended should include an explanation of the divergence from the formulary choice.

The definition stated that performance management is an overarching process by which organisations achieve desired outcomes; that is a little like stating a mathematical formula along the lines:

$a = f \times b$, where f is an unknown function of some sort.

As in the formula, the 'function', overarching process, needs a little further explanation to be of any use. The Department of Health in the *Priorities and Planning Framework* dealt with performance management, providing some of that explanation.[2] The document explains that local organisations are to have good monitoring systems in order to meet targets and that they will achieve those targets by taking appropriate corrective action if required. The statement starts to bring out the various elements of organisational performance management. To performance manage successfully, there need to be clear targets, information available on performance against those targets, a system of reviewing and action planning based on the information, and celebration when targets are achieved. To support these elements, there needs to be clear accountability and the empowerment of individuals and of teams to act when necessary.

The elements of performance management

The four elements listed merit further discussion before applying performance management to strategic medicines management. But a word of caution is warranted. Performance monitoring can too easily displace performance management. Performance indicators and benchmarking are important tools in performance management, but developing sophisticated measures of performance that are meaningful is not an end in itself. Taking performance management only that far would be a little like the captain of the *Titanic* being given all the information possible on the distance from the iceberg, his speed and so on, but doing nothing to change course. Perhaps a particular problem for pharmacists involved in performance managing regarding medicines is their scientific background and ability to concentrate on detail. Both of these are assets but could mean they focus on the minutiae of measurement and monitoring. The risk is that action to put things right is never initiated. If this is a fair analysis, then it is a strong reason to ensure that strategic medicines management is a multidisciplinary activity.

Setting targets

Taking performance management as an overarching process by which organisations achieve desired outcomes means that setting targets in line with these outcomes is vital. It may be that certain targets or even all targets are externally imposed. This has been the case in NHS organisations in recent years. To achieve the aims of *The New NHS: Modern,*

Dependable and *The NHS Plan*, clear targets and significant investment have been provided.[3,4] Targets have not been open to local negotiation or to test 'buy-in' but explicit and monitored publicly, with the star-rating system the most visible feature.[5] These targets have included maximum waiting time for elective surgery and a defined, increasing percentage of patients dealt with in under four hours on attending accident and emergency departments. Where targets are imposed externally, certain aspects of the target-setting process are redundant. However, even then, there are some features that remain the same. *The NHS Plan* itself was, of course, developed after very broad consultation with the public and professionals, so it could be argued that there was fundamental buy-in to the basic ideas.

Target setting is best informed by obtaining three views: internal, customer and external. The internal view is formed by looking at the vision and values of the organisation, and by seeking the views of staff. Another way of putting this is: 'What targets stem from the organisation's core purpose?' The customer view is to ask which targets should be set to ensure that service users have their needs met. Patients probably fit this description for strategic medicines management. The external view seeks to pick up targets that are set in national documents, by professional bodies or learned groups, as well as by peers.

Involving the organisation in target setting is a way of developing ownership and increasing the commitment of staff to the targets. Even where targets are provided, there still needs to be a process of developing buy-in. Gaining this commitment ought not to be along the lines: 'The NHS says we must achieve x and if you don't play your part you can leave!' Rather, it should be an exploration of why the target is important and how it can be made most relevant to the organisation. However, it would be naive to imply that there is no element of 'we have got to do it, because we have got to do it'.

Finding out what patients want can be achieved by both reactive and proactive methods. Learning from complaints has an important, although limited, role to play. Gaining information from patient surveys and from primary research can also help. Obtaining information is not easy. Focus groups and other methods may help, but are difficult to do well. It may be that membership and the members' council of NHS foundation trusts will provide a source of helpful advice on the needs of patients and service users.

Knowing what peers are doing or what their levels of performance are, should be more straightforward than being certain what patients want. Best practice and suggested standards will often make their way into national documents and improvement programmes. For other sources, interest groups of pharmacy organisations such as the Guild of Healthcare Pharmacists and the United Kingdom Clinical Pharmacy Association may be useful. Peer-reviewed and other journals for research-based and news articles can also be informative.

Benchmarking is a tool that can be used in a number of ways. It can contribute to performance measurement but it can also be used to inform target setting. The vision for medicines management in an organisation may be along the lines of 'making the most of medicines for patients by achieving best practice across the breadth of the service.' The best practice can be turned into specific targets by seeing what happens elsewhere and testing local practice against this benchmark. In a business-focused book, Zairi and Leonard explain benchmarking as the process of continuously checking ones own services, processes and products against the strongest competition – those known as world leaders in their fields.[6] They draw on Sun Tzu's *The Art of War* – know your enemy. The point is well made: if we are determined to do the best for our patients, we need to take seriously what that best can be. Roberts and Sharott apply this to pharmacy management: benchmarking 'allows managers to consider alternative ways of planning and delivering services based on the wider experience of others'.[7]

In setting targets for performance management it must be remembered that targets will drive performance. The consultancy firm TQM International Limited point out that it is vital that the right targets are set.[8] This seems quite obvious (and we will discuss measuring shortly), but targets are all too easily set because they are easy to measure, not because they are important. There is a parallel here to the old story about a little boy who lost his sixpence on a dark night while walking home across a field. A passer by asks him why he is searching the pavement. He explains his loss and, further, that it was dropped in the field, but that he is looking on the pavement because that's where the road lamp makes it possible to see. Targets should be set because they help achieve key objectives, not because they can be monitored easily.

The discussion has been of targets, but this is quite a broad term. 'Performance indicator' is a more precise term used in the NHS and beyond. Performance indicators are specific measures of economy, efficiency or activity. The term is used within the star-rating system already mentioned. Freeman provides a very helpful discussion of their use in the UK, focusing on some of their problems (gaming, short-termism and so on) and how their cautious use can be part of the overall assessment of how performance is going.[9] The performance indicator is the measure; the target is set that states what value or figure the perform-ance indicator is required to be for the organisation to declare it has achieved its goal.

Throughout the process of performance management, the basis of target setting should not be forgotten: what is to be achieved, by whom, by when? Lack of clarity here can make the whole process meaningless or lead to a situation where targets are simply not met.

Information on performance

Once clear, understood, measurable targets are set, there is a need for timely, accurate information on performance against those targets. The source and type of data will depend on the target. There may be simple dichotomous information – is the objective achieved or not. An example would be whether the board had approved a policy regarding the formu-lary or availability of medicines. The target may require continuous monitoring of a trend towards a specific endpoint, for example, the percentage of GP practices where the formulary has been integrated into the prescribing system. A third type of target is where a continuous measure to achieve a standard is required, for example, staying 1% within the budget set for spend on medicines or percentage of formu-lary compliance in an outpatient setting.

Key sources of information relevant to strategic medicines manage-ment will be PACT data, hospital prescribing systems (or for those without e-prescribing, pharmacy management computer systems), audits and other routinely collected data. The aim should be to have minimum effort in collection, accuracy, a shared understanding by all involved and access in a timely fashion. The point about a shared understanding is important. Disputes over accuracy, meaningfulness, relevance and interpretation can use much of the time and energy required for the next step – reviewing and acting. Getting the system right, correcting mistakes and being sure you do not act on misinformation are important, but this needs to be done 'quickly and quietly' behind the scenes rather than being the focus of attention of the whole organisation.

Review and action

This is possibly the part of performance management most easily forgot-ten and yet the most important. It might also be the hardest part, particularly if challenging rather than bland targets have been set. The way reviewing is approached will need to fit the organisation in terms of practical arrangements and style. What the targets are and how they are measured will also be relevant. Assuming the targets are organisational, rather than different for each team or locality, then access to monitoring data should be available to all. This may not always be appropriate and data that could be linked to individuals (prescribers or patients) require sensitive handling.

This 'passive availability' is only one part of the process. There needs to be appropriate face-to-face discussion of performance, backed up with written and electronic, but directed, information. Those who have a degree of management or clinical responsibility for the targets should be involved in the meetings.

For a PCT, the core team for performance review may be the prescribing lead, pharmacy lead and general manager, with reports to the board as well as to any medicines or therapeutic committee. Feedback to locality leads or senior partners in practices may also follow. For a hospitals trust, the group reviewing performance may be the therapeutic committee or a governance group.

Knowing how well the organisation is doing is only worthwhile if corrective action follows if needed. When an organisation has a dozen or so key targets and finds it is off course on several, then considerable effort may be required to improve matters. There may be sound explanations for divergence from targets and these could lead to adjustments being made. This luxury has not been available for trusts achieving their waiting time targets.

As with target setting, the action plans need to be clear. For example, who is doing what and over what timescale must be agreed and clearly stated to all. This approach to targets will almost certainly mean that managerial and some clinical effort will be diverted from all other actions to those delivering the key targets. This raises two important points. First, setting targets right and setting the right targets, are vital. Second, some aspects of any service will be difficult to set targets for – even if going beyond a narrow interpretation of performance indicators. The obsession with target achievement must therefore be moderated. Action to achieve a target should not entail failing to achieve other objectives or include actions that are contrary to the vision and values of the organisation.

Celebration

Good performance management must include celebrating success. For some targets there may only be a few key players; more usually many people both inside and outside the organisation will have contributed to target achievement. Their roles should be celebrated. Clearly, individual performance review can provide this in a focused way, but more general communication and publication of success is also warranted.

Celebration can also include some reflection. Why did things go well? What more could have been done on those targets nearly achieved? Were some targets unhelpful to the organisation's goals? Celebration is also a means of building support for the next steps or for the following year's targets.

Mentioning celebration could imply something else needs to happen if targets are not met. Prolonged failure to meet targets that really matter in an NHS organisation is likely to result in external intervention. This process will re-invigorate efforts to achieve targets. When things are not quite that bad, then some celebration will be appropriate and reflection on what more could be done undertaken. Re-visiting benchmarking work to see if others have shared similar problems or have developed new solutions would be helpful. If everyone has missed a key target there may be something wrong with the target or simply more time is needed.

The other factors

Accountability and empowerment are two factors that are worth examination. Accountability in this context is about being clear who has responsibility for the targets and action, as well as knowing to whom performance management reporting will be done. Being vague about who is responsible for what, is likely to lead to non-achievement of targets. This is more about who should take action than it is about fear of being held to account.

Empowerment of staff to manage their own performances, developing solutions to problems so that targets are met, is likely to be more successful than imposed performance management and solutions. 'Empowerment' has become a popular word in the NHS, but if commitment, rather than its use as a buzzword occurs, it is argued that results are improved and staff benefit.[10]

Applying performance management

Strategic medicines management has a number of features. In the introduction the definition used in this book is explained. In that context how does performance management play a part? Performance management should enable organisations to achieve the desired goals of good strategic medicines management. The process brings a discipline to the performance that results in a focus on delivery. This 'delivery' could be of change or of ongoing standards, as explained earlier. Strategic medicines management is not only about single organisation objectives; health communities, or prescribing patches, have shared responsibilities regarding new medicine entry, equity of access, reducing waste and so on. It was argued earlier that the way to deal with this in performance-management terms is to ensure that organisations have objectives that help to achieve the desired outcomes of the whole health community.

In England, the responsibility for performance management lies with strategic health authorities. Although medicines management themes have not featured obviously in NHS trust star ratings, they are present for primary care trusts. For all organisations, financial performance is a key responsibility and controlling medicine spend is an important feature.

For strategic medicines management, there may be process-related targets, as well as more outcome-based ones. The targets loosely described as outcomes-based may include outcomes in the sense of spend or volume of prescriptions, or be true outcomes related to health gain. Healthcare staff may feel more comfortable in dealing with a target that is along the lines of 'curing 95% of a certain disease' but, as with general NHS targets, they may need to be satisfied with targets such as 'reviewing 95% of patients taking more than four medicines'.

What targets are there?

Primary care

The NHS star rating for primary care trusts includes a number of targets that should be achieved.[11] Under 'access to quality services', there is an expectation that the proportion of atypical will rise. That is, the ratio of atypical to typical will increase year on year. This stems from the NICE guidance and relates to improved safety. A requirement to have recent audit data on the performance on the effective interventions for coronary heart disease is included in the improving health section. This is a measure of audit but it highlights interventions including medicines. Flu vaccination percentage rates are also included. The number of generic prescription items as a percentage of all prescription items excluding those for dressings and appliances is a further measure of performance. Prescribing rates of antibacterials and of benzodiazepines are both included under the service provision section. The aim here is to ensure that the problems associated with these two groups of medicines are minimised by ensuring appropriate use. Ratings on each indicator are available to the general public via the NHS website and rankings appear on overall trust performance, then for each indicator. The comparison is to average performance. Thus, Bassetlaw PCT is a three-star organisation for 2002–03 but performs significantly below average on the rate of atypical antipsychotic prescribing and at average for benzodiazepine and antibacterial prescribing.[12] Another three-star PCT (Central Suffolk) scores as average on atypical antipsychotics, above average on antibacterials and at significantly above average for benzodiazepines.[13] Such measures may feel rather focused on a part of the process, but can help form part of the target setting for strategic medicines management. A PCT may wish to see a set percentage improvement across all practices in one of these indicators or derive an action plan to achieve a shift.

There are many other requirements and demands on primary care organisations. The NPC document on responsibilities related to prescribing and medicines management gives a summary of the key targets and documents.[14] *Medicines and Older People* is emphasised as an important driver for action – medication reviews and gaining better help from pharmacists are highlighted.[15]

Further targets related to medicines management issues were included in the 2001 handbook for the NPC's medicines management collaborative programme. All targets have importance, but perhaps some fall in the medication management part of Figure I.2, rather than strategic medicines management.[16] In shortened form they were:

- percentage of requests for repeat scripts that were incomplete
- . percentage of patients receiving scripts without proper dosage instructions
- percentage of patients saying, when asked, that they had problems with the repeat system
- percentage of nursing home patients who have had a recent medicines review
- percentage improvement from baseline in locally agreed areas using health improvement outcomes or value for money measures
- percentage of practices who get timely discharge information on 90% of their patients.

Some results from the use of these targets can be seen described in the report on wave two of the collaborative on the NPC website.[17]

Although the star ratings and NPC collaboratives are both fairly recent, prescribing performance indicators that help target setting have been around for some time. The Audit Commission's document of primary care prescribing in 1994 provided some basic measures of good prescribing.[18] Other indicators of quality of prescribing can be developed and derived from national documents. Ensuring that funds are available for NICE implementation and that patients have access to medicines once a positive NICE appraisal is issued, are two areas for performance targets. What specific targets are set will depend on local position in respect of these or other national requirements. Focused action by the medicines management team to achieve and maintain success will be vital.

Hospital trusts

A specific set of targets relating to strategic medicines management in hospitals were issued in 2001 by the Department of Health.[19] This framework document identified six domains for trusts to ensure that systems or processes be in place:

- senior management involvement
- good use of financial information and control
- policies, including how new medicines are dealt with
- procurement
- the interface with primary care
- the influencing of prescribers.

Fitzpatrick reports how the West Midlands performed against this framework, with the first area of board involvement being weakest.[20] Not all of these areas have been included in this book's definition of strategic medicines management, but many are. Improving performance against these objectives will be a key part of local medicines management strategies.

The second round of the medicines management framework was launched in 2003.[21] The domains had changed a little and the document informed by *A Spoonful of Sugar* from the Audit Commission.[22] They were:

- senior management involvement
- information, finance and business planning
- medicines policy
- procurement
- designing services around patients – including patients' own medicines
- influencing prescribers and training
- managing risk.

Table 9.1 The Hospitals Medicine Management Collaborative NPC measures

Measure	What is sought
The number of patients saying yes when asked: Did you have problems with your medicines during your stay in hospital?	A reduction
The number of prescriptions referred back for clarification before dispensing	A reduction
The number of patients who have their discharge home delayed owing to problems with medicines	A reduction
The number of times a medicine is not available in time for the patient's next dose	A reduction
The number of acute hospital admissions where a documented medication history review is not undertaken within 24 hours of that admission	A reduction
The time taken from the request for an essential new medicine being made, to it being available for use	A reduction
The number of wards *not operating*	
use of patients' own medication	A reduction
self-medication scheme (where appropriate)	A reduction
dispensing for discharge (one-stop dispensing)	A reduction
The total number of non-formulary items dispensed	A reduction
The number of prescriptions that have not had a clinical review by a pharmacist at the point of dispensing	A reduction

The number of discharges from hospital where the following are *not* fully documented on the discharge summary:
    any changes in medication made during the admission
    the reasons for any changes
	A reduction

(Personal communication, NPC 2004)

Scores were reviewed by strategic health authorities and then action plans for organisations could be informed by the results.

The announcement in 2004 of the first and second waves of hospital trusts involved in the NPC's hospital medicines management collaborative opened the door to further possible measures and targets.[23] The initial measures that can act as performance indicators and hence be a basis for targets, were developed by an expert panel and are shown in Table 9.1.

The report on the uptake of NICE-approved cancer medicines deals with cancer networks, but each trust would need to check its own systems for ensuring access to medicines is given support.[24] A simple target of usage is not easily set – being in the mid-quartile of usage seems such a bland expectation. Audit may be the only way to develop a picture of how the organisation is performing, but the target of achieving access for patients within three months would appear reasonable.

Hospitals may also wish to develop targets relating to the clinical risks around medicines. Eliminating certain errors – intrathecal vinca alkaloid administration, intravenous bolus of potassium chloride solution – or achieving comprehensive reporting from all professions may be included.

As with primary care trusts, the detail of target setting will depend on local circumstances and position on these assessment frameworks.

Making it work locally

The process of target setting and implementing action to achieve them will require local leadership and a good deal of focus. Checking that the individual organisations targets do not clash with those of partners in the local health community will be important. The role of the prescribing committee across the patch will be central in this. Strategic medicines management has a history of organisations acting in their own interest, perhaps because of the way the rules were set, and much time has been taken to correct matters. The reduction in length of treatment on discharge is a good example, cut to save money for hospitals, then lots of pressure to restore to a reasonable length to allow original pack dispensing. This example shows how performance management can be both good and bad. The imperative in the 1980s and 1990s was to see balanced hospital budgets – no matter what – so good performance-managing organisations achieved this. But the target was not the best one in terms of continuity of patient care. The message is get the right targets and then the effort of delivery will be worthwhile.

References

1. Stephens M. Performance management – delivering a successful hospital pharmacy service. *Pharm Manage* 20: 9–12, 2004.
2. Department of Health. *Priorities and Planning Framework*. London: DH, 2002.
3. Department of Health. *The New NHS: Modern, Dependable*. London: The Stationery Office, 1997.
4. Department of Health. *The NHS Plan: a Plan for Investment, a Plan for Reform*. Norwich: The Stationery Office, 2000.
5. NHS Star ratings explanation. http://www.nhs.uk/england/aboutTheNHS/starRatings/default.cmsx (accessed 15 December 2004).
6. Zairi M, Leonard P. *Practical Benchmarking: The Complete Guide*. London: Chapman & Hall, 1994.
7. Roberts P, Sharrot P. Managing services. In Stephens M, ed. *Hospital Pharmacy*. London: Pharmaceutical Press, 2003.

8. TQM International Limited. *Performance Measurement Workbook.* Frodsham: TQM International, 1996.

9. Freeman T. Using performance indicators to improve health care quality in the public sector, a review of the literature. *Health Serv Manage Res* 2002; 15: 126–137.

10. Miller D, ed. *Leading Empowered Organisations.* Leeds: Creative Health Care Management/Centre for the Development of Nursing Policies and Practice, 2002.

11. NHS Star ratings targets for PCTs. http://nww.nhs.uk/Root/StarRatings/PCTPIS.htm#KeyTargets (now unavailable; see http://www.nhs.uk/england/aboutTheNHS/starRatings/default.cmsx; accessed 15 December 2004).

12. NHS Star ratings performance, Bassetlaw PCT. http://nww.nhs.uk/Root/StarRatings/Trust.asp?orgcode=5ET&Type=pct (now unavailable; see http://www.nhs.uk/england/aboutTheNHS/starRatings/default.cmsx; accessed 15 December 2004).

13. NHS Star ratings performance, Central Suffolk PCT. http://nww.nhs.uk/Root/StarRatings/Trust.asp?orgcode=5JT&Type=pct (now unavailable; see http://www.nhs.uk/england/aboutTheNHS/starRatings/default.cmsx; accessed 15 December 2004).

14. National Prescribing Centre. *PCT Responsibilities Around Prescribing and Medicines Management.* Liverpool: NPC, 2003.

15. Department of Health. *Medicines and Older People, Implementing Medicines Related Aspects of the NSF for Older People.* London: DH, 2001.

16. National Prescribing Centre. *Collaborative Medicines Management Services Programme Handbook.* Liverpool: NPC, 2001.

17. National Prescribing Centre. Medicines management collaborative, wave two review. http://www.npc.co.uk/mms/Web_Dev/Extras/wave2_review.pdf (accessed 8 December 2004).

18. Audit Commission. *A Prescription for Improvement: Towards More Rational Prescribing in General Practice.* London: HMSO, 1994.

19. Department of Health. *The Performance Management of Medicines Management in NHS Hospitals.* London: DH, 2001.

20. Fitzpatrick R. Strategic medicines management. In Stephens M, ed. *Hospital Pharmacy.* London: Pharmaceutical Press, 2003.

21. Department of Health. Medicines management in NHS Trusts: hospital medicines management framework. http://www.dh.gov.uk/Publications AndStatistics/Publications/PublicationsPolicyAndGuidance/Publications PolicyAndGuidanceArticle/fs/en?CONTENT_ID=4072184&chk=RuVaBK (accessed 15 December 2004).

22. Audit Commission. *A Spoonful of Sugar: Medicines Management in NHS Hospitals.* London: Audit Commission, 2001.

23. National Prescribing Centre. Hospital medicines management collaborative. http://www.npc.co.uk/mms/hmmc/measures.htm (accessed 15 December 2004).

24. Department of Health. Cancer medicines uptake. http://www.dh.gov.uk/PublicationsandStatistics/Publications/PublicationsPolicyAndGuidance/PublicationsPolicyAndGuidancearticle/fs/en?CONTENT_ID=4083901&chk=vkfy2d (accessed 16 June 2004)

10

The research agenda

An issue that has cropped up several times in this book has been the lack of clear, high-quality evidence that demonstrates the value of the interventions used within strategic medicines management. There is, perhaps, some inevitability in this. Medicines management describes a wide range of complex activity, with many interacting strands. Trying to identify the specific benefit of, say, a formulary in isolation from the impact of clinical pharmacy services, the level of medical support or the type of prescribing system used, is a difficult task. Some of the interventions have been around a long time and were introduced when practice research was not well-established; thus the opportunity to assess the impact is possibly lost. However, there are many questions that can still be investigated and, as services develop, so too can the research agenda, informing those changes and identifying the benefits when changes are made. This chapter explores some of the areas where research is required and the possible methods that could be used.

Medicines management and pharmacy practice research

The introductory chapter details the emergence of the term 'medicines management'. Even before this, work to explore the impact pharmacy services can have on the use of medicines had been established. The Nuffield report noted some progress was being made to explore the benefits of pharmacy input, although outcomes-based research was lacking and the volume and scope were limited.[1] The *Way Forward* circulars in 1988 provided an impetus for clinical pharmacy services but also gave a boost to pharmacy practice research.[2] Further support was given by the Pharmacy Practice Research Enterprise Scheme.[3] At this time there was a blossoming of various streams of practice research based around academic practice units, often linking university departments and practitioners. Mays reported a considerable amount of work being undertaken, but noted that there was a lack of consistently high-quality work, and what existed was of a descriptive nature.[4]

During the late 1990s, the Pharmaceutical Society provided a number of reports to push forward pharmacy practice research. A detailed report encouraging a culture of research for all pharmacists, with a smaller proportion actively involved in research was issued in 1997.[5] More focused papers on issues such as self-care research, therapy and pharmacy, and on the profession followed.[6–8] The key messages from these documents were the need to address important healthcare priorities, the need to produce good research outputs, the need for a culture of evaluation and the need for adequate financial support for practice research.

In 2000 Alexander reported progress made in practice research.[9] She reviewed the practice research at the British Pharmaceutical Conference that year, including oral and poster presentations. Seventy-six papers were considered; several were randomised controlled trials, but quasi-experimental design, surveys and qualitative methods were also present. A wide range of subjects were included, with 'prescribing support' and 'risk management' covering the topics that seem to fall into the area of strategic medicines management research. Alexander commented that methods used tended to be more robust than had been the case a few years earlier, but that work remained small-scale.

Examining the details of practice research presented at the 2003 conference shows a similar range of methods employed and, of the 96 items, about five appear to fall into the strategic medicines management field.[10]

A recent report by Child, Cantrill and Cooke described the methods for finding evidence of the effectiveness of hospital pharmacy services.[11] They also describe some of the issues and opportunities for current and future practice research. Their paper categorises the research identified in searches, and 'strategic medicines management' heads the list with 76 references found from 1980 onwards. They list clinical audit, drug-use review and formulary services in their definition. They restricted their work to UK hospital pharmacy practice. They concluded that there is still much to do and that some areas are considerably under-researched. Better coordination was seen as necessary.

University departments now often have active research programmes in the field of medicines management. Strategic medicines management, pharmaceutical care and other themes are included. Keele's department of medicines management includes themes on pharmacoepidemiology, medicines policy, concordance, and substance misuse, on the research section of its website.[12] Jointly with Aberdeen and Nottingham universities, Keele is evaluating the Pharmaceutical

Services Negotiating Committee's medicines management project – which is focused at an individual care level. The Drug Usage and Pharmacy Practice academic group based in Manchester University has a research profile encompassing medicines and pharmacy practice. Themes include prescribing, health economics, local pharmaceutical services evaluation and management of minor ailments.[13] The School of Pharmacy in London is example of an academic department where good links have been developed with hospitals; areas of work include evaluating pharmacy services, health technology assessment and consumer perspectives on medicines.[14] Other schools of pharmacy have similar, practice-based research programmes and operational research related to medicines forms elements of other academic department programmes.

Practice research is encouraged by the various pharmaceutical organisations in the UK. Opportunities to disseminate work are provided, via oral presentation and by poster, for example, by the United Kingdom Clinical Pharmacy Association and by the Guild of Healthcare Pharmacists. The Faculty of Prescribing and Medicines Management of the College of Pharmacy Practice produced a draft practice research strategy in March 2003.[15] Its aims were to encourage the entire faculty membership to participate in practice research and to ensure that research was on a multiprofessional basis. The opportunities for research listed in the document included patient specific work, which is indeed vital, but also work under the definition used here of strategic medicines management.

Watson and McCloughan report the support and encouragement given to practice research, and other aspects of practice and research, by the Scottish School of Primary Care.[16] Their emphasis is on ensuring that skills are developed in primary care to use research, be involved with research, actively participate in research and lead research.

There appear to have been significant steps taken to encourage research in the area of medicines management, including the strategic elements. There remain many opportunities to carry this work forward, but these need to be using robust methods, be multiprofessional in nature and be on a larger scale than has often been the case.

The NHS context

Just as there have been significant changes in NHS organisational arrangements and in NHS funding flows, so have there been changes in the area of NHS research and development. In March 2000, the Department of Health published a document on the funding arrangements for research and development in the 'new NHS'.[17] The document summarised the approach to research:

- for basic and strategic research, the department contributes to the Research Councils' strategies and supports NHS costs of hosting research
- for public health and health service research and development, the department leads with a contribution from other organisations.

Medicines management research tends to fall into the latter category – although this does not mean such work stems only from the department's programme. Two streams of funding were identified: NHS priorities and needs research, and development funding and NHS support for science. The former includes work on service delivery, which is where strategic medicines management research and development sits. Research was to be of a high standard and to support national priorities.

The NHS Service Delivery Organisation National Research and Development Programme was set up at the same time as the funding document was launched. It aims to consolidate and develop the evidence base relating to the organisation, management and delivery of health services. Information on its work can be found on its website: www.sdo.lshtm.ac.uk. One funded opportunity of pertinence to medicines management was the request for proposals to examine issues of concordance, adherence and compliance in medicine taking. A scoping exercise was sought, with a target date to complete by late 2004. The request for bids noted the complexity of the topic and the need to involve several disciplines and perspectives. This is an important point, relevant to most strategic medicines management research.

In 2001, the *Research Governance Framework for Health and Social Care* was published by the Department of Health.[18] It identified the need for high standards within research, to ensure quality outputs and to protect the patient. This approach mirrored the clinical governance agenda for general healthcare. The framework document points to a number of pieces of legislation already present, for example, the Data Protection Act 1998. Standards of financial probity are set for research, which are already expected in NHS organisations, being covered by corporate governance arrangements. One implication of this is a need to be clear on the costs and funding sources for research undertaken in the NHS. The need for ethical review of research was restated in the framework. For Wales and Scotland similar frameworks have also been issued.[19,20]

Ethics

Strategic medicines management practice research is subject to ethical review in the same way as clinical trials of new medicines. The purpose of ethical review is to protect the patients, public and other subjects, including NHS staff. Strategic medicines management research and development may involve introducing or withholding a specific intervention from a group of patients or a population. The ethical review will examine if this is reasonable – is there equipoise between the two experimental arms, or is one approach proven to be safer. Safety issues will be considered – are subjects exposed to unreasonable risks or even to small risks with no useful purpose? Issues of confidentiality and of appropriate informed consent will be reviewed. Projects that seek information from healthcarers will be required to demonstrate that coercive participation is avoided.

Where a project is undertaken within an organisation or on a local basis, a local ethics research committee will need to give a favourable opinion. For larger scale projects involving organisations across a wider geography, a multicentre ethics committee opinion is required. Details of these arrangements can be found on the Central Office for Research Ethics Committees (COREC) website: www.corec.org.uk. The website includes details of when to apply for advice from an NHS research ethics committee, with the relevant clauses for strategic medicine management being where patients are included, where carers of NHS patients are included, where NHS premises or facilities are used or where NHS staff are included because of their professional roles.[21,22]

What are the research questions?

National guidance

The existence of NICE and SMC guidance raises a number of issues of interest to researchers. The World Health Organization's work on NICE addressed some issues, and other work on thresholds has been undertaken.[23,24] The question of how NICE guidance impacts on resource allocation locally is important. Does a pending NICE appraisal mean that access is delayed compared with the historic trend? This involves some retrospective analysis and is subject to confounding, but merits examination. For items not addressed in NICE programmes, is there a delay in use? How does the availability of NPC documents affect use of these not-NICE-reviewed products? Access to therapies supported by

NICE guidance has been the subject of political enquiry and has received media attention. Where there are delays, these could be due to a variety of reasons. Some technologies require complex delivery; others are more straightforward. There are opportunities to examine the geographical uptake of NICE therapies and to explore the reasons for delay. An important, although complex, area for research would be to examine the characteristics of organisations and health communities where there is rapid and effective implementation of NICE guidance. Have such communities used the model suggested in the NPC document? Do they perform well in other aspects of healthcare delivery? An example would be to map the uptake of a selection of NICE appraisals against the performance ratings of a cluster of organisations. The report from the Department of Health on uptake of cancer medicines across English cancer networks, as discussed in Chapter 1, is a possible starting point for such work.[25]

Chapter 1 also notes the important move to empower patients and to involve them in healthcare decisions and planning. The research and development agenda here ranges from a simple mapping of how such activities are being introduced, to exploring the most effective way to engage the public and patients in strategic medicines management issues. Although much has been done in terms of individual patient issues – compliance, concordance, adherence and patient empowerment – there is little on how involvement at a higher level is best organised or what effects such input has.

Local organisational approaches

Following on from overall lay involvement, the specific area of patient and public involvement with area and organisational DTC is a subject for study. There is much we do not know. What benefits ensue from such involvement? How is lay or patient involvement best delivered? Are there any dangers to the decision-making process that emerge from patient input? Do decisions differ between DTCs that have lay input from those that do not? The final question here may be particularly interesting, but particularly hard as almost no two DTCs have similar membership. There are questions that can be informed by research in this general area, rather than only learning from specific, DTC-based work; thus any NHS group or committee seeking effective lay input may allow learning on the best way for inclusion of patients and the public.

The more general question of what are the best organisational arrangements for DTCs, would also benefit from research and development work. A model was proposed earlier in this book, of an area DTC with organisational DTCs implementing guidance from the former. Is this a model that works effectively? Comparing different models around the UK, in terms of their outputs and impact on medicines use, may enable a best practice model to emerge. Research could lead to the conclusion that many different models can work effectively, so long as certain key elements exist. Work by the NPC has sought to explore this in the past.[26]

Assuming a shared definition of an effective area DTC is achieved, it would also be interesting to map implementation of NICE guidance to effectiveness of DTC. Are the two linked? It may be that where DTC arrangements fail, other systems come into play to ensure that guidance is implemented.

Formularies

The use of formularies is now commonplace, even if randomised controlled trials on their impact is lacking. They form one part of the strategic medicines management framework, so probably do not now need a major research programme focusing on them in isolation. That said, there are issues of design, access, use of e-versions and so on, that merit attention. Examining the cost-effectiveness of the production and maintenance of different models – single versions for a whole health community, simple list versus guideline collation – may still require attention.

Managing entry

Where local decisions are needed regarding new medicines or preferred choice of established medicines, considerable work is required on critical appraisal, decision making, prioritisation and dissemination. The research and development agenda here is rich. How well are critical appraisal reviews undertaken for local DTCs and organisations? What skills are needed to prepare such documents? Does the workforce have these skills? What is the best way to develop skills to ensure that informed decisions are taken?

Decision making in public organisations, use of evidence and ways of disseminating decisions do not just apply to medicines. As with other aspects of strategic medicines management, this area can be informed by other streams of work.

The subject of safety in managing the entry of medicines has been raised by the National Patient Safety Agency.[27] How this is best achieved, what impact is made and how decisions are affected is another theme for medicines management research.

Work to compare what medicines are chosen as first line and how decisions are reached across different organisations in different areas would provide an insight into managed entry issues. There may be justifiable variation, or concerns on process could emerge.

Health economics

Work mentioned in Chapter 5 includes a study on whether health economic literature was used to inform decision making. This work may be worth repeating in the light of the profile that cost-effectiveness has in NICE appraisals. The ability for DTCs and medicines managers to access and use health economic data is of interest – perhaps particularly to those who can provide support to improve use of such work. The issue of equity requires attention too. Do DTCs take account of equity, in its broadest sense, while coming to prioritisation decisions? Do professionals and the public see this as an important factor in deciding on medicines use?

Systematic approaches

So far in the discussion, individual issues have been considered. As Chapter 7 describes, strategic medicines management should be seen as a whole-systems approach, an approach that seeks to make the most of medicines. Taken in this way, the need for research and development at systems level becomes apparent. North Staffordshire and Southampton reviewed their systems and made changes to improve medicines management.[28,29] In neither case was a planned research programme intended, although in both reports some analysis of impact was included. In each case the organisation acted as its own control, over time. The Audit Commission used the North Staffordshire work to inform their *Spoonful of Sugar* in which they highlighted the variation in performance in medicines management across hospitals in England and Wales.[30] They drew out features that should lead to good performance; these, along with items in the performance management frameworks, can inform the research agenda. Five key questions were derived to answer the overall question of whether the trust provides an effective medicines management service. These were:

- Is there effective control over medicines expenditure?
- Is staffing adequate for the services that should be provided?
- Is the use of pharmacy staff cost-effective?
- Do pharmacy staff devote enough time to direct patient care?
- Has the service introduced processes in line with accepted practice?

Of course, these are audit issues, not research questions, but they raise a range of issues that merit attention. Intertrust comparison of these issues, exploring the impact that changes in any or all parameters make to patient care and spend are worth study.

Other issues, such as use of directorate pharmacists, how prescribers are best supported and influenced, and how best to deliver induction regarding safety of medicines also require investigation.

Similarly in primary care, there needs to be an exploration of the best ways to organise and deliver strategic medicines management support at practice and organisational level. In those PCTs consistently delivering prescribing indicators and balancing their prescribing budgets, what are the organisational features or characteristics that bring success? Are those characteristics unique to each organisation or is there an opportunity to learn and spread success? The Faculty of Medicines Management included the effectiveness of pharmacy advisers as an area for research and development attention.[15] How important is leadership in these issues? This has been raised for clinical care; similar work is perhaps needed for strategic medicines management. Similarly, the effectiveness of team working may impact on medicines use and implementation of prescribing policy. This merits attention.

Budgets and performance management

Chapter 8 highlights the substantial information available in primary care to examine spend on medicines. This allows interorganisation and interpractice comparisons. Such information informs the research subjects mentioned above. Approaches to budget setting, systems for monitoring and control – if not already covered above – can also form the basis for research questions. There may well be no one best way to undertake these responsibilities, but there may be lessons to learn by examining the benefits and disbenefits of different methods.

Similarly there may be more or fewer effective ways of performance managing medicines management. Exploring what works and what problems occur in a systematic, rather than anecdotal, way could improve overall performance as lessons are learnt collectively.

The research and development process

The discussion so far has been of research ideas and subject areas. Effective research and development in strategic medicines management depends on a number of steps. Asking an appropriate question, framed in a meaningful way, is an important first step. Clarity at this stage can prevent problems as the methods are chosen and developed. The same issues arise here as are discussed in Chapter 4 regarding clinical trials. The question may arise from an issue in practice, where the professional wants to know something, looks in the literature and finds a gap. There may be several stages of refining the question so that it becomes answerable within the likely timescale and resources. If the literature has not been visited, this should be done. It may be that the research already exists or the answer can be pieced together from what is already in the literature.

Once a well-defined question has been posed, a suitable methodology needs to be chosen. Although randomised controlled trials are considered the method most likely to provide a 'correct answer', not all questions lend themselves to this approach. Smith discusses the various methodologies for evaluating services in her text on research methods.[31] She points out that RCTs have been described as inappropriate for practice research because they are not generalisable – too narrow a selection of subjects and so on – because blinding participants to the intervention becomes very difficult, and because outcomes and endpoints are often not clear in such research, hence comparing interventions becomes difficult. RCTs may not be the appropriate methodology for the question. For example, qualitative methods can address issues around the preferences, beliefs or attitudes of patients. Crombie and Davies give an example of the answers that qualitative research touches that RCT methodology simply cannot reach: 'It is very easy to discover that some patients fail to keep their appointments at outpatient clinics, but uncovering the reasons for this can be much more taxing.'[32] Qualitative methods can help to reveal the whys and hows of situations and services. Such methods include direct observation, interviews and focus groups. The term 'operations research' has been used to describe another set of techniques that may be useful in strategic medicines management. It involves the exploration of the way healthcare is organised and delivered, providing insight into complex systems where there is uncertainty in the interrelationship of several factors. The approach usually involves developing a model of the service or system under investigation.

Revisiting the question, examining the literature and then considering each of the available research methodologies should allow a plan for the practice research to be developed. Seeking funding, ensuring that data collection methods are feasible, finding a researcher and gaining a favourable ethical opinion, all take time. Planning, with realistic timescales, is of great importance. Appropriate advice from relevant experts – statisticians, qualitative researchers, health economists and so on – will be invaluable throughout the process.

Data analysis will be a key part of the research, whichever method is used. A well-planned approach that suits the methodology is required. This may involve fairly simple tally charts, more complex statistical packages or, for qualitative work, content analysis based on transcripts or recorded interviews. As with clinical trials, bias can be brought in at this stage just as in design.

Interpreting the results, drawing conclusions and then dissemination need to complete the research. Care needs to be taken in interpretation, to avoid making causal links that are not supported, or simply drawing unjustified conclusions. Poor interpretation can lead to otherwise good research being ignored. Various safeguards can be used. Research should have predefined questions; post-hoc analysis of unexpected questions should be undertaken very cautiously. Objectivity and cautious interpretation of results, avoiding inflated claims, are other safeguards. Although it is important to use an appropriate statistical test, showing statistical significance is not the same as showing that a difference matters. The issue of the importance of the results – 'What should we do about them?' – should be included in any discussion.

Dissemination of results should be an aim of all researchers. There are a wide range of peer-reviewed journals, exhibitions for posters and conferences for oral communication. If knowledge is to be developed and practice taken forward, research findings need to be shared. Perhaps academics are better at this than practising healthcarers. Feeling that research was small scale or that it was not rigorous can be reasons not to publish, which emphasises the need to get this right. Selecting a method of dissemination that fits the type of work undertaken and will reach the right audience is essential. Ideally, the target publication should be considered before the write up is started.

Table 10.1 provides some examples of issues, research questions and possible methodologies relevant to strategic medicines management. Smith describes various examples of research that would fit into this theme, using the heading 'initiatives to influence prescribing.'[31] Use of routine prescribing data (PACT data for example), is seen as an appropriate tool to assess the impact of such services, but other quantitative and qualitative approaches are also described.

Table 10.1 Strategic medicines management research: possible methodologies

Area of interest	Questions	Possible methodology
Do area DTCs work?	How are area DTCs organised?	Survey
	How do area DTCs make decisions?	Survey
		Focus group
		Observational study
	Do area DTC decisions influence medicine usage?	Quasi-experimental design comparing different communities
		Routine data collection
Are directorate and practice pharmacists useful?	Do the benefits derived from the work of directorate pharmacists outweigh the costs?	Health economic modelling using cost–benefit approach
	Do practice pharmacists increase uptake of specific clinical guidelines?	'Clinical trial' approach with radomised allocation of pharmacists to practices
	What are the perceived benefits of a practice pharmacist from a practice staff perspective?	Semistructured interviews
		Focus group

DTC = drug and therapeutic committee.

Funding

The need to fund NHS based research was mentioned earlier. This can be a sticking point for practitioners, although there are a range of funding sources available. The Royal Pharmaceutical Society provides two sorts of practice research awards: the Galen award and the Linstead Fellowship. The former is made annually and is up to £10,000; £40,000 is available via the latter scheme and is earmarked for community pharmacy research. Additionally, various bursaries are available.[33,34] Other pharmaceutical organisations, such as the Guild of Healthcare Pharmacists and the United Kingdom Clinical Pharmacy Association, offer awards to support and develop research.

The NHS Research Capacity Steering Group has developed a number of research training award schemes and, as mentioned above, the Department of Health commissions research in line with NHS priorities. The Medical Research Council has also supported healthcare research, where strategic medicines management research would sit. There are also a whole host of charitable sources for research; these are often focused on specific diseases. Thus the National Asthma Campaign or the Stroke Association will provide funding for research, although strategic medicines management projects may not easily sit in one area.

There are a number of aspects to obtaining research and development funds. Once the research idea and draft plan have been developed, the potential researcher should identify possible research fund sources. The topic of research will help direct to the suitable source. It is important to clarify the research interests of the potential funding bodies, to tailor the application appropriately. The basics of ensuring that the information requested is provided, and correct completion of the forms, must not be overlooked. A research funder will want to be clear on the purpose of the research and the expected benefits. They will also want to know that their monies will produce results. Inevitably, seeking research grants will be a process requiring persistence. Several initial rebuffs should not lead to abandoning a good idea. Gaining advice from experienced researchers or seeking collaboration with researchers who have track records will strengthen any proposal.

Conclusion

Research related to strategic medicines management has an important part to play in developing good medicines use. Although not everyone will be a fulltime researcher, everyone should be using evidence to provide the best possible service in an effective way. Many pharmacists, pharmacy technicians and other healthcare professionals are needed to contribute in some way to research, whether in idea generation, data collection, active research or dissemination and review. There are many organisations and academic institutes willing and ready to support those in practice to be involved in research. There are also opportunities to develop research skills via taught courses. Web-based resources, such as RDDirect are available to aid the would-be researcher.[35] The introduction of some of the early strategic medicines management initiatives may have had scanty high-quality evidence. The healthcare community should ensure that this does not occur with ideas currently emerging. Those that do develop new services and undertake good evaluations need to disseminate their findings, opening them up to scrutiny, to allow good practice to flourish.

References

1. Clucas K (Chair). *Pharmacy: The Report of a Committee of Inquiry Appointed by the Nuffield Foundation.* London: The Nuffield Foundation, 1986.
2. Department of Health. *The Way Forward for Hospital Pharmaceutical Services* HC 88(54). London: DH, 1988. Also WHC 88(66) (Wales) 1988 and 1988 (GEN) 32 for Scotland 1988.
3. Pharmacy Practice Research. *The Pharmacy Practice Research Enterprise Scheme: a Resource Document.* Manchester: Pharmacy Practice Research, 1990.
4. Mays N. *Health Services Research in Pharmacy: a Critical Personal Review.* Manchester: Pharmacy Practice Research Resource Centre, 1994.
5. The Royal Pharmaceutical Society of Great Britain with King's Fund Policy Institute. *A New Age for Pharmacy Practice Research. Promoting Evidence-Based Practice in Pharmacy, the Report of the Pharmacy Practice Research and Development Task Force.* London: RPSGB, 1997.
6. The Royal Pharmaceutical Society of Great Britain. *Practice Research: Setting the Research Agenda, Self Care and Pharmacy.* London: RPSGB, 1998.
7. The Royal Pharmaceutical Society of Great Britain. *Practice Research: Setting the Research Agenda, Drug Therapy and Pharmacy.* London: RPSGB, 1998.
8. The Royal Pharmaceutical Society of Great Britain. *Practice Research: Setting the Research Agenda, Pharmacy and the Profession.* London: RPSGB, 2001.
9. Alexander A. Designs and methods becoming 'more robust'. *Pharm J* 2000; 265: 406–410.
10. British Pharmaceutical Conference, 2003. *Int J Pharm Pract* Pharmacy Practice Research suppl. http://www.pjonline.com/IJPP/bpc2003/index.html (accessed 8 December 2004).
11. Child D, Cantrill J, Cooke J. The effectiveness of hospital pharmacy in the UK: methodology for finding the evidence. *Pharm World Sci* 2004; 26: 44–51.
12. Department of Medicines Management, Keele University. http://www. keele.ac.uk/depts/mm/Research/ragend.htm (accessed 13 December 2005).
13. Manchester University Drug Usage and Pharmacy Practice Group. http://www.pharmacy.manchester.ac.uk/Research/DrugUsage (accessed 15 December 2004).
14. University of London School of Pharmacy. http://www.ulsop.ac.uk/depts/ practice&policy/practice&policy.htm (accessed 15 December 2004).
15. Asghar M. *Practice Research Strategy, Working Draft 1.* Coventry: College of Pharmacy Practice Faculty of Prescribing and Medicines Management, 2003.
16. Watson M, McCloughlan L. How the Scottish School of Primary Care can help pharmacists. *Pharm J* 2004; 272: 63–64.
17. Department of Health. *Research and Development for a First Class Service, Research and Development Funding in the New NHS.* London: DH, 2000.
18. Department of Health. *Research Governance Framework for Health and Social Care.* London: DH, 2001.
19. Wales Office of Research and Development for Health and Social Care. *Research Governance Framework for Health and Social Care in Wales.* Cardiff: National Assembly for Wales, 2003.

20. Scottish Executive Health Department. *Research Governance Framework for Health and Social Care in Scotland*. Edinburgh: Scottish Executive, 2001.

21. Central Office for Research Ethics Committees. http://www.corec.org.uk/applicants/help/faqs.htm#a (accessed 17 December 2004).

22. Department of Health. Governance arrangements for NHS Research Ethics Committees. http://www.dh.gov.uk/PublicationsAndStatistics/Publications/PublicationsPolicyAndGuidance/PublicationsPolicyAndGuidanceArticle/fs/en?CONTENT_ID=4005727&chk=CncpyR (accessed 17 December 2004).

23. World Health Organization. *Technology Appraisal Programme of the National Institute of Clinical Excellence. A Review by WHO. June–July 2003*. Copenhagen: WHO, 2003.

24. Towse A, Pritchard C, Devlin N. *Cost-effectiveness Thresholds: Economic and Ethical Issues*. London: King's Fund, OHE, 2002.

25. Cancer medicines uptake. http://www.dh.gov.uk/PublicationsandStatistics/Publications/PublicationsPolicyAndGuidance/PublicationsPolicyAndGuidancearticle/fs/en?CONTENT_ID=4083901&chk=vkfy2d (accessed 16 June 2004).

26. National Prescribing Centre. *Area Prescribing Committees – Monitoring Effectiveness in the Modern NHS, a Guide to Good Practice*. Liverpool: NPC, 2000.

27. Department of Health. *Building a Safer NHS for Patients: Improving Medication Safety*. London: DH, 2004.

28. Fitzpatrick R, Mucklow J, Fillingham D. A comprehensive system for managing medicines in secondary care. *Pharm J* 2001; 266: 585–588.

29. Stephens M, Tomlin M, Mitchell R. Managing medicines: the optimising drug value approach. *Hosp Pharm* 2000; 7: 256–259.

30. Audit Commission. *A Spoonful of Sugar: Medicines Management in NHS Hospitals*. London: Audit Commission, 2001.

31. Smith F. *Research Methods in Pharmacy Practice*. London: Pharmaceutical Press, 2002.

32. Crombie I, Davies H. *Research in Health Care*. Chichester: Wiley, 1996.

33. Anon. Pharmacy practice: investing in research and securing the future. *Pharm J* 2003; 270: 34–35.

34. Anon. Pharmacists invited to apply for practice research funding under 2004 awards and bursaries scheme. *Pharm J* 2004; 272: 68.

35. RDDirect website. http://www.rddirect.org.uk (accessed 8 December 2004).

Index

absolute risk reduction, 93
access to evidence, 87–88
access to therapy, 1, 144
  equity in decision-making, 103–104
  evidence-based approach, 76
  formularies impact, 53, 54, 56, 65, 74
  legal aspects, 157–159
  marginal utility, 102
  NICE guidance implementation, 13, 14–15, 17
  Northern Ireland, 19
  research approaches, 199–200
  restrictions on new medicines, 74, 94
  Scotland, 18–19
accountability, 187
  performance management, 181, 182
Accounts Commission, 171
activated protein C, 33
adherence, 103, 200
  formularies use, 48, 50, 52, 59–60
  to guidelines, 133, 134–135, 139
adverse events, xiii, 17, 104, 128, 137
  impact of formulary use, 53, 54, 65
  new medicines, 65–66, 76
  Phase I clinical studies, 68
  reporting, 39, 69
advertising, 64
affordability, 74, 75, 94, 130
  restricted access to medicines, 159
age, sex and temporary-resident-originated
     prescribing units (ASTRO-PU), 168, 169
age-related decision making, 20
All Wales Medicine Strategy Group, 171
All Wales Prescribing Advisory Group, 171
allocative efficiency, 100–101, 117
Alzheimer's disease, 15, 110, 111
angina guidelines, 135, 136
antacids, 4
antibiotics, 54, 55, 104, 169, 173, 188, 189
  guidelines, 135
    impact on resistance, 136
  prophylaxis, 138
anticholinesterases, 15
anticoagulant guidelines, 126–127
antidepressants, 66
antiepilepsy drugs, 9
antifungal agents, 173
antiplatelet agents, 54, 80, 93
anti-tumour necrosis factor therapy (anti-TNF),
    14, 19
appraisal of evidence *see* critical appraisal
aspirin, 8, 12, 93
asthma guidelines, 124, 125, 127, 135, 136

atypical antipsychotics, 12, 54, 138, 188, 189
audit, 125, 156
  cancer medicines access, 191
  directorate pharmacists, 156
  guidelines implementation, 133
  NICE guidance compliance, 17
  non-formulary medicines prescribing, 157
  prescribing decisions, 155
Audit Commission, xix, xxi, 32, 145, 202
  formularies, 47, 48, 52, 57
  prescribing, 166, 169, 170, 190
average costs, 101, 102

back pain guidelines, 124, 125
benchmarking, 184, 187
benefits, 100, 144
  economic analyses, 111–112
  marginal, 101, 113
  measures, 106, 112
benoxaprofen, 65–66
benzodiazepines, 4, 170, 188, 189
bias, 83, 86, 111, 205
blobbogram (Forest plot), 80, 81
Bolam v. *Friern Hospital Management
    Committee*, 137
Boolean logic, 87–88
breast cancer, 18
British National Formulary, 64
  non-prescribable items, 4
budget management, 163–178
  'payment by results', 175–177
  primary care, 166–172
    active interventions, 169–170
    monitoring, 168
  research approaches, 203
  secondary care *see* hospitals
budget overspends, 163
budget planning, 159
  expected medicine developments
    information sources, 163–164
    list compilation, 165
  for future years' budgets, 165–166
  medicine-spend growth estimation, 165
  NICE developments funding, 166
  primary care, 165, 168

cancer care
  chemotherapy, 138
  guidelines, 135
  drug and therapeutic committees (DTCs), 33,
    34
  National Service Framework, 21

cancer care – *cont.*
  networks, 33, 37, 191, 200
cancer medicines, 15, 100, 172, 176, 191, 200
  cost of new drugs, 64
carboplatin, 109
carcinogenicity, 68
case control studies, 86
case reports, 86
case series, 86
case studies, 86
CENTRAL, 88
cervical cytology, 124
change management, 132
children
  National Service Framework, 21
  safety of antidepressants, 66
chlorpromazine, 64
cisplatin, 64
Citizens' Council, 9
clinical audit *see* audit
clinical freedom, 122
clinical governance, 121, 132, 157, 168
clinical guidelines *see* guidelines
clinical pharmacy, xiv, xv, xxi, xxii, 153
Clinical Resource Efficiency Support Team
    (CREST), 19
  Drugs Advisory Group, 19
Clinical Standards Board for Scotland, 132
Cochrane Central Register of Controlled Trials,
    88, 130
The Cochrane Database of Systematic Reviews,
    88
cohort studies, 86
College of Pharmacy Practice, Faculty of
    Prescribing and Medicines Management,
    xx–xxi
combination products, 4
Commission for Health Improvement, 121
Commission for Patient and Public Involvement
    in Health, 35
commissioning, 175, 176
communication skills, 41
community pharmacists, 170
comparative studies, 86
  effectiveness of new medicines, 69
compassionate use, 69, 73–74
compensation claims, 128
complaints, 17, 128, 183
compliance, 3, 200
  formulary use, 52
concordance, 2, 171, 200
confidence intervals, 85
confounding, 86, 111
consultant pharmacists, 156
continuous ambulatory peritoneal dialysis, 5
contracting, 115
controls assurance programme, xvi
coronary heart disease, 20
correlation studies, 86
cost shifting, 5–6, 32, 150
  shared care arrangements, 151
cost-benefit analysis, 105, 109–110, 111

formulary use, 56
  output measures, 112
  societal perspective, 110
cost-benefit issues, 94
cost-consequence analysis, 105, 116
cost-effectiveness, 74, 75, 100
  formularies, 56–57
  NICE appraisals, 11–12, 14
  restricted access to medicines, 159
cost-effectiveness analysis, 104, 105, 106, 111,
    116
  output measures, 112
cost-minimisation analysis, 105
cost-utility analysis, 105, 106–109, 111,
    115–116
  output measures, 112, 116
  perspective issues, 110
costs, xiii, xvii, xxiv, xxv, 100, 144
  average, 101, 102
  direct, 111–112
  drug and therapeutic committee (DTC)
    purposes, 26, 27
  economic analyses appraisal, 111–112
  formularies development/impact, 45, 46, 52,
    53, 55–56, 60, 144
  electronic prescribing systems, 58–59
  fundholder prescribing impact, 6–7
  guidelines impact, 124, 126, 128, 135, 136
  indirect, 111, 112
  intangible, 112
  marginal, 101, 102
  new medicines, 64, 65, 94
  North Staffordshire medicines management
    system, 149
  prescribing analysis and cost (PACT) data, 167
  prescribing incentive schemes, 7, 169
  Southampton optimising drug value project,
    146
  tangible, 112
  see also budget management
critical appraisal, 88–91, 92, 160
  drug and therapeutic committee activities, 41
  economic analyses, 110–113, 117
  guidelines development, 130–131
  medicines information, 153
  meta-analyses, 90
  randomised controlled trials, 90–91
  sponsorship issues, 89, 91
  systematic reviews, 89–90
critical care, 176
  networks, 33
Cumbria (North) Medicines Management
    Group, 32, 36
cyclosporin, 5

database searching, 87–88
Derbyshire (North) Priorities and Clinical
    Effectiveness Forum, 32, 36
devolution, 2, 29
diabetes
  ketoacidosis, 138
  National Service Framework, 21

direct-to-consumer drug promotions, 64
directorates
  hospital budget management, 172
  pharmacists, 155–156, 203
discharge medicines, 6, 146, 165, 192
discounting, 112–113
dosage efficiency, 170
doxorubicin, 15, 64
drug and therapeutic committees (DTCs),
    25–43, 86, 155, 160, 201
  access to information, 92–93
  area model (health communities), 35–37
  functions, 40
  budget management, 173, 174
  economic analyses appraisal, 110–111
  equity in decision-making, 103–104
  expected medicine developments appraisal,
    164
  formularies development, 46
  guidance on medicines, 39, 41
    guidelines development, 124
    guidelines implementation, 138, 139
    restriction of access, 157, 159
  historical background, 26–33
  meetings, 42
  membership, 41–42
  minor decisions, 41
  monitoring impact, 42–43
  network working, 33–34
  North Staffordshire Medicines Management
    Group, 148
  NPC good practice guide, 30, 31, 34
  organisational, 40, 42
  patient/public representation, 34–35, 42, 200
  presentation of evidence, 92–94
  primary care prescribing subgroups, 31–32
  purposes, 26–27, 32–33, 37–41
  research approaches, 200–201, 202
  shared care arrangements, 150, 151
  Southampton optimising drug value project,
    146
  task allocation approaches, 38–39
Drug Usage and Pharmacy Practice group, 197
DrugInfoZone, 153

e-formulary, 58–59
economic analyses, 100, 104–110, 117
  attached to randomised controlled trials, 114
  critical appraisal, 110–113, 117
  discounting, 112–113
  evidence base, 111
  generalisability/local application, 113
  margins analysis, 113
  perspective issues (whose valuation),
    110–111
  sensitivity analysis, 113, 114
economic models, 114–115
economics
  definitions, 99
  inputs (costs), 100
  margins, 101, 102, 103
  outputs (benefits), 100

  measures, 106, 112
  see also health economics
effectiveness, 74, 75, 94, 117
efficacy, 74, 94
  Phase II clinical studies, 68
efficiency, 100, 103
  allocative, 100–101, 117
  technical, 100
elderly people
  annual medicines review, 20
  medicines dispensing/administration, 20
  National Service Framework, 20
  prescribing indicators, 168
electronic databases, 87
electronic learning packages, 155
electronic prescribing analysis and cost (PACT)
    data, 167
electronic prescribing systems, 58–59, 155, 172,
    173
  decision support systems, 58, 59
EMBASE, 87, 130
EQ-5D, 107
equity, 103
errors
  elimination targets, 192
  monitoring, 39
erythropoietin, 5
  shared care arrangements, 150–151
escitalopram, 18
ethical review of research, 198, 199
ethics research committees, 199
EuroQuol health state score, 107, 108
evidence hierarchy, 77, 78, 83, 85, 86
  guidelines development, 123, 130
evidence-based medicine, 13, 64, 76–95, 144
  access to evidence, 87–88
  appraisal of evidence, 88–91, 92
  clarity of questions examined, 92
  formularies use, 53, 57–58
  guidelines design, 123
  presentation of evidence, 91–94
  restriction of access to medicines, 159
  type of evidence, 77–86
expert opinion, 86, 92, 109, 160
  economic models, 115
  guidelines development, 123, 131
expert patient, 34
explanatory trials, 75
external validity (generalisability), 83, 89

flu vaccination, 188
fluoxetine, 71
focus groups, 183, 204
Forest plot (blobbogram), 80, 81
formularies, 45–60, 117, 121, 143, 155,
    156–157, 171
  adherence, 52, 59–60
    compulsion, 48, 50
  character/style, 48
  community/intended users, 48, 51
  coverage/therapeutic areas, 48, 49–50
  definitions, 45, 47

formularies – *cont.*
  design, 48–51
  development/update of list, 52
  educative role, 59
  electronic systems (e-formulary), 58–59
  feedback to prescribers, 52–53, 55–56
  guidelines incorporation, 48, 49, 59, 124
  historical background, 45–47
  impact, 52–57, 74
    evidence base, 53, 57–58
    prescribing costs, 52, 53, 55–56, 60, 144
    prescribing quality, 52, 53–55, 60
  non-formulary medicines prescribing, 148,
    157
  primary care/hospital joint working, 48, 51
  research approaches, 201
fundholding, 6–7, 28, 56, 169
funding, 5–8, 74
  cancer services, 33
funnel plot, 80–81, 82

Galen award, 206
general medical services (GMS) funds, 5
general practice
  electronic prescribing systems, 58
  formularies, 51
    adherence, 60
    development, 46, 47
    hospital care joint working, 48, 51
    prescribing quality impact, 54
  prescribing analysis and cost (PACT) data,
    167
  prescribing budgets, 6–7, 168
  shared care arrangements, 150, 151
  see also primary care
general practitioners (GPs)
  drug and therapeutic committee (DTC)
    membership, 26, 28
  legal duty to prescribe, 157–158
general sales products, 8
generalisability (external validity), 83, 89
  economic analyses, 113
generic prescribing, 69, 71, 165, 169, 170, 171,
    188
  impact of formulary use, 56
Glasgow medicines management approach, 160
glatiramer acetate, 10–11
GP Prescribing Support, 30
growth hormone, 5, 167
guidelines, 121–139, 143
  access at point of prescribing, 132
  adherence, 133, 134–135, 139
  audit criteria, 131
  clinicial attitudes, 135–136
  content, 125–126
  criticisms, 13
  definitions, 121–123
  desirable attributes, 126
  development, 13, 122–123, 155, 156
    process, 127, 128–131
  development group, 130
  dissemination, 131–132

divergence, 122, 137
evidence base, 123, 127, 130
formulary design, 48, 49, 59
grading of recommendations, 123, 131
historical background, 124–125
impact, 133–137
  patient outcome, 136
implementation, 132–133
legal aspects, 137
local, 128, 130, 131, 132, 134, 138–139
national, 134, 135, 137, 138, 139
National Institute for Clinical Excellence
    (NICE), 9, 12–13
  compliance audit, 17
North Staffordshire new medicines
    introduction system, 148
patient empowerment, 134, 135
prescribing decisions, 155
purpose, 122, 123, 124, 128, 134
strategic medicines management, 124
subject selection, 128
see also shared care guidelines

head injury, 9
health communities, 35–37, 181
health economics, 41, 99–117, 130
  applications, 114–116
  concepts, 100–104
  economic analyses, 104–110
  guidelines impact, 126
  research approaches, 202
health gains
  discounting, 112–113
  measures, 106, 112, 116
    monetary valuation, 109
health-related quality of life, 106
  economic models, 115
  scoring systems, 106–108
healthcare resource groups (HRGs), 176, 177
  national average price, 175, 176
hip prostheses, 9
historical policy changes, 2–8
horizon scanning, 71–74, 153, 156, 159
  budget planning, 163–166
  drug and therapeutic committees (DTCs), 29
  medicines information documents, 72, 73
horizontal equity, 103
hospital and community health services
    (HCHS) funds, 5
hospital pharmacy committees *see* drug and
    therapeutic committees (DTCs)
hospitals, 29
  budget management, 172–175
    chief pharmacist's role, 172, 173
    devolved budgets, 172–173
    feedback to clinicians, 174
    monitoring, 173, 174
    overspend correction, 174–175
    prescriptions dispensed in community,
      173–174
    unexpected prescribing, 173
  budget overspends, 163

budget planning, 165
computerised stock control systems, 172, 173
directorate pharmacists, 155–156
drug and therapeutic committees (DTCs), 26, 27–28, 173, 174
electronic prescribing systems, 172, 173
formularies, 51, 156–157
 adherence, 59
 character/style, 48–49
 compulsion in adherence, 50–51
 development, 45, 46, 47
 prescribing costs impact, 55
 prescribing quality impact, 53, 54
 primary care joint working, 48, 51
funding allocation changes, 5–6
guidelines implementation, 138, 139
health economics in decision-making, 116
induction for junior doctors, 154
influencing prescribing, 154–155
medicines management targets, 190–192
performance review, 186
restriction of access to treatment, 158
hypercholesterolaemia, 135
hypokalaemia, 138

indicative prescribing budgets, 6, 7
information access, 87–88
insulin, 64
interferon beta, 115, 158
 NICE guidance, 10–11
internal validity, 83, 89
interventional procedure guidance, 9

laxatives, 4
legal aspects
 guidelines, 137
 restriction of access to medicines, 157–159
length of supply
 budget management, 170
 discharge prescribing, 192
 prescription charge strategies, 4
life cycle of medicines, 67–71
limited list, 4–5
 substitution effect, 4
Linstead Fellowship, 206
literature searching, 78–79, 92, 130
 electronic databases, 87–88
local organisational approaches, 25–43
London New Drugs Group, 29–30, 36, 88
Lothian Formulary, 46
Low Income Scheme Index, 169

macroeconomics, 99
managed entry, 63–95
 costs impact, 64, 65
 horizon scanning, 71–74
 management of medicines, 73–74
  restriction of access, 74
 patient safety, 65
 planning, 71, 72, 73
 prescribing responsibility, 66–67
 research approaches, 201–202

marginal analysis, 113, 117
marginal benefits, 101, 113
 diminishing utility, 103
marginal costs, 101, 102
market authorisation, 63, 69, 71, 74, 94
market launch, 69
marketing, 64–65, 69
 approach to guidelines implementation, 132–133
Medical Research Council research funding, 207
medicine development process, 67–68
 adapted versions development, 69
 market authorisation, 69
 market launch, 69
 patent expiry response, 67, 69, 71
 Phase I clinical studies, 68
 Phase II clinical studies, 68, 71
 Phase III clinical trials, 68–69, 71
 Phase IV postmarketing trials, 69
Medicines Act, 63
Medicines and Healthcare Products Regulatory Agency (MHRA), 63, 66
medicines information services, 71, 72, 73, 88, 115, 153–154
 expected medicines developments, 163–164
MEDLINE, 87, 130
mental health
 guidelines, 135
 National Service Framework, 21
meta-analyses, 78, 79–80, 83, 123
 appraisal, 90
microeconomics, 99
Midland Therapeutic Review and Advisory Committee (MTRAC), 28, 30, 34, 36, 149, 150
Misuse of Drugs Act, 63
monitoring therapy, xiv–xv
multiple myeloma, 18
multiple sclerosis, 10–11, 115, 158
myocardial infarct
 post-infarct thrombolysis, 20
 prophylaxis, 9, 12

named patient use, 69
National Health Service (NHS)
 foundation trusts, 29, 42, 176
 funding flows, 5–8, 32, 175
  'payment by results', 175–177
  unified approach to hospital/primary care, 5–6, 166
 post-1997 organisational changes, 29
 research/development funding, 197–198, 206–207
National Horizon Scanning Centre (NHSC), 71, 72
National Institute for Clinical Excellence (NICE), 8–18, 28, 29, 30, 33, 71, 72, 115, 121
 Citizens' Council, 9
 cost-effectiveness thresholds, 11–12, 14
 criticisms, 11, 13

National Institute for Clinical Excellence – *cont.*
  evidence hierarchy, 77, 78, 83, 85, 86
  Guideline Review Panels, 13
  guidelines, 12–13, 138
    development, 123, 125, 128, 131
    funding under 'payment by results', 176,
      177
    research approaches, 199–200
  implementation of guidance, 12, 14–16, 33
  National Collaborating Centres, 13
  performance appraisal, 13–16
  response procedure, 16–18
    audit, 17
    local impact assessment, 17
    resources, 18, 166
  structure, 8–9
  technology appraisals, 9–12, 14
    appeals, 9, 10
    assessment reports, 9
    cost-utility analyses, 109, 116
    expected developments information,
      163–164
    process of production, 9
    response to negative appraisals, 17
National Prescribing Centre (NPC), xv, xx
  horizon scanning, 71
  medicine management targets
    hospital trusts, 191
    primary care, 189
  medicines development information, 163
  medicines information documents, 72, 73
  prescribing strategies, 170
National Service Frameworks, 19–21
  prescribing costs impact, 169
  roles, 19–20
negligence claims, 137
  scheme for trusts, 128
network working (CNST), 33–34
New Drugs in Clinical Development, 72
New Drugs Online, 72
new medicines, 28, 121
  adverse effects, 65–66, 76
    reporting, 69
  affordability, 74, 75
  compassionate use, 69, 73–74
  cost-effectiveness, 74, 75
  decision-making for access, 74, 94
  development process, 67–68
  effectiveness, 74, 75
    comparative, 69
  efficacy, 74
  evidence-based decisions, 76–95
  expected developments information, 163–164
  formulary use, 53, 54, 56
  funding, 30–31
    under 'payment by results', 176, 177
  hospital budget management, 175
  impact assessment for budget planning, 164
  managed entry, 63, 64, 65
  marginal utility, 64, 65
  marketing, 64–65
  'me-too' agents, 74

modified formulations, 74
North Staffordshire introduction system, 148
novel agents, 74
prescribing responsibility, 66–67
restriction of access, 157, 158, 159
shared care arrangements, 151
specialist prescribing, 5–6
withdrawal, 66, 71
The New NHS – Modern, Dependable, 5, 19,
  33, 47, 103, 182–183
NHS *see* National Health Service
The NHS Plan, 34, 35, 67, 183
NHS Quality Improvement Scotland (NHS
  QIS), 18
NICE *see* National Institute for Clinical
  Excellence
night sedation, 169
non-randomised studies, 85–86
non-steroidal anti-inflammatory drugs, 54, 55
North Staffordshire medicines management
  system, 147–149, 160, 202
Northamptonshire prescribing project group,
  32
Northern Ireland, 19
  formularies development, 46
null hypothesis, 84
number needed to harm (NNH), 93
number needed to treat (NNT), 82, 93
nurse-led services, 20

odds ratio, 80, 82
On the Horizon, Future Medicines, 72
On the Horizon, Rapid Review, 72
operations research, 204
opportunity cost, 99
oral contraceptives, 3
outpatient prescriptions, 6
ovarian cancer, 9, 72
over-the-counter medicines, 8

p value (statisitical significance), 84–85
packaging, 66
paclitaxel, 109, 158
PACT data *see* prescribing analysis and cost
  (PACT) data
paracetamol, 69
paramedic-delivered care, 20
patents expiry, 67, 69, 71, 165, 171
paternalisnm, 1, 2
patient advocacy and liaison services, 34
patient decision-making, 122, 158, 171
patient empowerment, 1, 2
  guidelines, 134, 135
patient involvement, 160
  drug and therapeutic committees (DTCs),
    34–35, 42, 200
  feedback, 17
  performance target setting, 183
  research approaches, 200
patient-focused healthcare, xiv, xvi, xxii, 1
'patients' own drug' schemes, 60, 146
'payment by results', 175–177

healthcare resource groups (HRGs), 175, 176, 177
reference costs, 176
tariff prices, 176
penicillin, 64
performance indicators, 184–185, 189
performance management, xviii–xix, 181–192
accountability, 187
action planning, 182, 186
application to strategic medicines management, 187–188
celebrating success, 186–187
definition, 181
drug and therapeutic committees (DTCs), 42–43
hospital budget management, 174
information sources, 185
monitoring, 182, 184, 186
research approaches, 203
review, 185–186
staff empowerment, 187
targets, 181, 182–185, 186, 187
person trade-off, 108
pharmaceutical care, xiv, xvii, xxi, xxii, 121, 196
Pharmaceutical Services Negotiating Committee, 196–197
pharmacoeconomics, 99
pharmacy practice research, 195–197
Phase I clinical studies, 68
Phase II clinical studies, 68, 71, 74
Phase III clinical trials, 68–69, 71, 74, 75
power of trial, 84, 85
Practice Formulary, 46
practice pharmacists, 155–156
pragmatic trials, 75, 111
pre-payment certificates, 4
prescribing
committees *see* drug and therapeutic committees (DTCs)
decisions, 152–156
clinical audit, 156
education/training, 154–155
medicines information services, 153–154
strategic medicines management, 153, 154
dosage efficiency, 170
incentive schemes, 7, 169
indicators, 168, 171
Low Income Scheme Index, 169
therapeutic group measures, 169
weightings, 168–169
length of supply, 170, 192
repeat, 170, 171
restriction of access to medicines, 156–160
reviews, 6
shifting from hospital to primary care, 28, 32, 150
prescribing analysis and cost (PACT) data, 167, 185, 205
Prescribing Indicators National Group, 168
Prescribing Outlook, 72, 163, 164
Prescribing Support Unit, 167, 168, 169

prescribing unit (PU), 168
prescription charges, 2–4, 8
effectiveness model, 3
exemptions, 2, 3
impact on demand, 3–4
Prescription Pricing Authority, 167, 168
primary care
budget management, 166–172
funding allocation changes, 5–6
medicines management targets, 188–190
prescribing, 155, 158, 170
DTC subgroups, 31–32
research approaches, 203
see also general practice
Primary Care Trust Resource Limits, 168
primary care trusts (PCTs), 29, 47
budget management, 166–172
inter-practice/organisation comparisons, 168
monitoring, 168
practice-based pharmacist advice, 170
repeat prescribing, 170–171
budget planning, 165, 168
expected medicine developments appraisal, 164
guidelines development, 139
incentive schemes, 7
NICE guidance implementation, 12
performance review, 186
PRODIGY, 58–59
product launch-related rapid appraisals, 29
prostate cancer, 18
provider–purchaser split, 27
publication bias, 81

qualitative research, 204
quality of life *see* health-related quality of life
quality of prescribing
formularies impact, 52, 53–55, 60
prescribing analysis and cost (PACT) data, 167
prescribing incentive schemes, 7, 169
prescribing indicators, 168
Prescribing Support Unit activities, 167–168
primary care targets, 189–190
quality-adjusted life year (QALY), 106, 116
criticisms, 108–109
health-related quality of life scoring system, 106–108
person trade-off approach, 108
standard gamble approach, 108
time trade-off approach, 108
quasi-experimental studies, 85–86
pharmacy practice research, 196

randomised controlled trials, 83–85, 123, 204
appraisal, 90–91
attached economic analyses, 114
bias, 83
confidence intervals, 85
confounding, 83–84
external validity (generalisability), 83

randomised controlled trials – *cont.*
  internal validity, 83
  pharmacy practice research, 196
  sample size, 85
  statistical analysis, 84–85
  statistical significance (*p* value), 84–85
recombinant human deoxyribonuclease, 5
relative risk, 80, 82
repeat prescribing, 170, 171
research, 195–207
  budget management, 203
  data analysis, 205
  dissemination of results, 205
  ethical review, 198, 199
  formularies, 57–58, 201
  funding, 206–207
  health economics, 202
  interpretation of results, 205
  local organisational approaches, 200–201
  managed entry, 201–202
  methodology, 204, 206
  national guidance, 199–200
  NHS funding, 197–198
  performance management, 203
  pharmacy practice, 195–197
  planning, 205
  process, 204–206
  systematic medicines management
    approaches, 202–203
*Research Governance Framework for Health
    and Social Care*, 198
resource allocation, 10, 160
  allocative efficiency, 100–101
  legal issues, 159
  local drug and therapeutic committees
    (DTCs), 39, 41
resource scarcity principle, 99
restricted access to medicines, 156–160
restricted use prescribing, 28
rheumatoid arthritis, 14, 19
riluzole, 149
risk management, 42
risks, xiii, xvi, xix, xxiv, xxv, 64, 128,
    160–161
risperidone, 5
Rosser-Kind index, 106, 107, 108, 109

safety, 65, 160
  managed entry of new medicines, 65, 202
  research project review, 199
sample size, 85
Saving Lives: Our Healthier Nation, 103
schizophrenia, 12
Scotland
  budget planning, 164
  formulary use impact, 55
  medicines advice, 18–19, 33
  NICE guidance information dissemination,
    18
  primary care prescribing budgets, 171
  primary care/hospital joint formularies, 48
Scottish Intercollegiate Guidelines Network
    (SIGN), 123, 128, 131

Scottish Medicines Consortium (SMC), 18, 19,
    33, 199–200
secondary care *see* hospitals
selection bias, 80, 81–82
self-care, 2
sensitivity analysis, 113, 114
  economic models, 115
shared care guidelines, 149–152
  development, 152
  patient-centred approach, 151
  review, 151
shared care prescribing, 28
simvastatin, 171
societal change, 1–2
Southampton Drug Finance Group, 31, 146
Southampton optimising drug value project,
    145–147, 160, 202
specialist prescribing, 5–6
specific therapeutic group age/sex-related-
    prescribing units (STAR-PU), 169
standard gamble approach, 108
Standing Group on Health Technology
    Assessment, 29
statins, 8, 12, 51, 52, 84, 85, 100, 138, 165,
    167, 171
  guidelines, 135
statistical analysis, 84
statistical significance (*p* value), 84–85
steroid inhalers, 167
strategic health authorities, 29, 36, 37, 188
strategic medicines management
  definitions, xxi, xxii–xxiii
  importance, xxiv–xxv
substitution effect, 4
systematic medicines management approaches,
    143–161
  research, 202–203
systematic reviews, 77–83, 88, 123, 130
  appraisal, 89–90
  evidence assessment, 79
  evidence summation, 79
  interpretation of findings, 80, 82
  literature search, 78–79
  meta-analysis, 78, 79–80, 83
  problems, 82
  selection bias, 80, 81–82

tacrolimus, 150
targets
  clinical errors elimination, 192
  medicines management, 188
    hospital trusts, 190–192
    local focus of delivery, 192
    primary care, 188–190
  monitoring performance, 185, 186
  performance management, 181, 182–185,
    186, 187
  prolonged failure to achieve, 187
  setting, 182–185
    benchmarking, 184
    internal views, 183
    patient involvement, 183
taxanes, 9

technical efficiency, 100
technology appraisals *see* National Institute for
    Clinical Excellence (NICE)
teratogenicity, 68
therapeutic substitution, 4, 145–146
time trade-off approach, 108
topotecan, 64
toxicology, 68
tricyclic antidepressants, 80
type 1 error, 84
type 2 error, 84

UK Medicines Information Group (UKMi), 72,
    73, 153
  medicines development information, 163
  Training Workbook, 87
unlicensed medicines, 94
unwanted medicines, 177–178

validity, 83, 89
venlafaxine, 66

vertical equity, 103
vision, 144

Wales, prescribing indicators, 171
Wales Task and Finish Group, 32
waste prevention, 177
  formularies use, 60
  'patients' own medicine' scheme, 146
  repeat prescribing, 170
Wessex evaluation committee, 28, 29
Wessex Formulist, 49
Westminster Hospital Formulary, 45–46
willingness to pay, 109–110
wisdom teeth removal, 9
withdrawal of medicines, 66, 71

yellow card scheme, 69

z-drugs, 9
zanamivir, 11
zoledronic acid, 18